Health Information Technology Standards

Philip A. Smith

Tim Benson
Series Editor

Making Computerized
Provider Order Entry Work

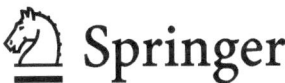 Springer

Philip A. Smith
Sanford
Florida
USA

ISBN 978-1-4471-4242-3   ISBN 978-1-4471-4243-0   (eBook)
DOI 10.1007/978-1-4471-4243-0
Springer London Heidelberg New York Dordrecht

Library of Congress Control Number: 2012949279

Printed on acid-free paper

Springer is part of Springer Science+Business Media (www.springer.com)

Foreword

It is better to be a dog in a peaceful time than be a man
in a chaotic period.
Ancient Chinese Proverb

Many believe the above proverb to be the source of the oft-repeated phrase, "may you live in interesting times." There is little doubt that in American healthcare at the time of this writing (spring 2012) we are living through interesting times.

The last 30 years of American healthcare has witnessed remarkable technological advances in the fields of imaging, pharmacotherapeutics, and surgical interventions, to name a few. However, simultaneously, U.S. healthcare has come under scrutiny as society pays more attention to the dissociation between the cost of healthcare and its demonstrable benefits to the American public, at least as compared with the rest of the civilized world.[1] One answer to this problem has been the pursuit of information technology as a structural answer to both improved efficiency and effectiveness of healthcare delivery in our country.

The president signed The Health Information Technology for Economic and Clinical Health (HITECH) Act, enacted as part of the American Recovery and Reinvestment Act of 2009, into law on February 17, 2009, to promote the adoption and meaningful use of certified health information technology. Since that time, there has been a marked increase in acquisition and efforts at implementation of electronic health records (EHRs) in large, medium, and small healthcare settings in our country. This informatics transformation of American healthcare will have ramifications for all aspects of the practice of medicine in our country for decades to come.

This book is an essential manual to getting that transformation right.

Dr. Phil Smith, the Chief Medical Information Officer for the Adventist Health System, and his team have demonstrated that implementation of computerized

---

[1] Squires DA. The U.S. health system in perspective: a comparison of twelve industrialized nations. Issue Brief (Commonw Fund). 2001;16:1–14.

patient order entry (CPOE) in 26 hospitals in 28 months[2] can be accomplished effectively and safely realizing the benefits of these new technologies in the daily practice of medicine.

Dr. Smith steps you through the vision, management, lessons learned and metrics that every CMIO, CIO, and CMO should know to achieve successful acquisition, configuration, and implementation of EHRs. The contents include examples and experience from the 26 hospital Adventist system as well as lessons from leaders in applied medical informatics throughout the United States.

These lessons have been learned from first-hand experience in system configuration, design, and importantly, lessons of leadership in healthcare information technology (HIT) management that are essential to guiding medical professionals through the challenging transitions from early adoption to effective benefits realization.

This comprehensive guide elaborates on elements of the successful transition to EHR adoption in detail including:

1. Leadership skills
2. Project management from the CMIOs perspective
3. Course correction in dealing with the inevitable resistance to change
4. Building a successful team and maintaining motivation.

However, beyond the comprehensive guidance Dr. Smith provides in this book, he reveals the caring insight to the "diagnosis and treatment" of modern healthcare informatics challenges that stems directly from his tradition as a physician and educator. The astute reader and student of this book should note the balance the author strikes between firm leadership and guidance, and the clinician's empathy and partnering skills to achieve the greater goal.

In these times of rapid change and growth in American healthcare informatics, this book stands as an important work to advise, enhance, and sometimes comfort the HIT leader as he or she navigates this essential transformation in American healthcare.

May 2012   William F. Bria, M.D.

---

[2] How 26 hospitals deployed e-order systems in 28 months. 2011. http://www.computerworld.com/s/article/9222681/How_26_hospitals_deployed_e_order_systems_in_28_months.

Preface

If I have seen a little further it is by standing on the shoulders of Giants.
–Sir Isaac Newton

Why should you read this book? Maybe you are planning a single hospital implementation of Computerized Provider Order Entry (CPOE) and want to pick up a few pearls. Perhaps you are with a large health system and are tackling a new project affecting all or most of your facilities. Alternatively, perhaps you want to assess as to what level of fool would tackle a project to rollout CPOE to 25 community hospitals, "big bang" over 28 months. The day I am writing this Introduction (August 2, 2011), our 26th hospital (yes, 26th) went live on house-wide CPOE, less than 25 months after our first CPOE pilot. In addition, our hospital physicians are all using CPOE with a company-wide average of less than 13 % verbal/telephone orders.

This book is about the process of making a complex project like this, or any other CPOE project, a reality. It is not the work of one person, but rather requires a team, leadership, clear vision, dedication, commitment, external drivers, experience, and the tireless work of those before us in this industry, who have paved the way with both successes and failure. Only by standing on the shoulders of the giants can we see beyond ourselves and achieve big goals. I like to sum it up humorously with a principle that has guided me in this project: "Do what has been shown to work in the past, and don't do what has been shown not to work."

This book is not a scientific reference guide into medical informatics, but rather a practical guide to visioning and executing successful automation of physician workflow in hospitals. This is not a book on theory or a summary of research studies in the field. Much smarter persons than I in the field have contributed the research and efforts to bring us through the last 30 years from the first CPOE system to the commercially supported systems of today. We all are indebted to them. There will be points in this book where I challenge conventional "wisdom" in the area of implementing CPOE. In the end, I hope that my peers will see this as an opportunity for dialogue and further study.

I once heard a motivational speaker tell a story about a wise executive who was quite successful at running his company.

> An employee asked, "How is it that you have been so successful at your business?" The executive answered, "I find it important to only make good decisions!" The employee then asked, "How did you find a way to only make good decisions?" "Oh, that was simple," answered the executive. "Early in my career, I made lots of bad decisions."

Throughout the book, I will be sharing hard lessons-learned and guide you through the early warning signs that will help you avoid the pitfalls. Unlike the wise executive above, I continue to make the occasional bad decision and learn from my mistakes. As systems progress, and the regulatory environments change, there will be new challenges and opportunities that will confront you in your efforts to automate physician workflow. However, there are principles such as vision, leadership, project management, and change management that will always need your attention for project success.[3]

Moreover, I would like to set the book up with a little prologue, so you will know a little more about the author and the team, how we came to tackle system-wide CPOE more aggressively than we might have otherwise. I hope this provides some useful context to these teachings in this book. My journey was not through traditional medical informatics training, but rather through a series of eclectic events. So my apologies up front to my many colleagues who are more scholarly in the field. Your contributions to the industry have been many and great, and I thank you for your passion into designing better systems and constructs for our future end-users.

My journey in medical informatics began in November 1993 when I converted my family practice office in New Port Richey, Florida, from paper to an electronic medical record (EMR). That first year, I found myself more productive and more profitable, and really caught the bug. Back in 1993, using an off-the-shelf EMR, I was keeping electronic problem lists, medication histories, allergies and reminders. Pharmacists were amazed that patients arrived with printed prescriptions and medication safety information. And patients who lived in Florida only during the winter (we refer to as "snowbirds") returned north each spring with a printed summary of care that today we would call a continuity of care document (CCD).

What was particularly useful to learn was the power of information in transforming care even within a single office of two physicians at that time. Though not particularly related to CPOE, a brief summary of some of these may yield some clues about my early passion for the EMR:

> We quickly learned that we had 76 phone calls a day into the office and that over half we had seen in the office in the prior 48 h. Of this latter half, the process typically was that the patient would call the receptionist (front-office staff), who would then transfer the call to the nurse (back-office staff), who would then take a detailed message and promise to call the patient back after speaking with the

---

[3] I strongly encourage physicians in the field of informatics to join AMDIS, the Association of Medical Directors of Information Systems. Their conferences and discussion groups at www. amdis.org are a priceless resource, and we encourage you to join.

doctor. Then the nurse would catch the appropriate doctor between patients, and jointly we would attempt to reconstruct what occurred at the prior visit, since prior to the EMR the dictation of the visit was typically pending at that time. Once the doctor devised a plan, the nurse would attempt to call the patient back (and this was before the popularity of cell phones) and relay the physician's advice. Overall, it often took an hour or two to close the loop as well as our nurse spending about 8–12 min per call and often longer.

We instituted a practice that each day the physicians would indicate patients on our schedule that our office nurse would call the following morning between 8 and 9 AM. These patients were either work-ins (i.e., sick and worked into the schedule acutely) or patients on whom we started new medications or treatments. Because the encounter visit was in the EMR, as well as structured and clear, the nurse could quickly call each patient proactively and inquire, "How are you feeling and do you any questions or concerns?" The patients loved this service and saw us as a team that cared for them. Moreover, the time the nurse spent per patient was typically 1–2 min, freeing up much time and effort.

The second opportunity involved patient flow and our ability to design a better schedule for our patients. Each physician had about 10,000 active patients. We would see about six work-ins daily in addition to our pre-scheduled appointments. Through electronic scheduling we were better able to devise a schedule that not only allowed us to see the walk-ins daily but stay close to our scheduled time with our planned patients for that day. For us, we built a modified-wave schedule, which had six appointment slots per hour – three at the top of the hour, two at 20 min after the hour, and one at 40 min after the hour. This allowed us to stay on time even though patients sometimes arrived later for their appointments. Each hour, we left one slot that was open and we could only schedule after 3 PM the prior day. As a result, we had a work-in slot for every hour, and patients soon learned that we could see them the same day if sick. When there were open slots, we used these to complete insurance inquiries or other paperwork. An unintended, but positive, consequence of this was that patients rarely called us after-hours (i.e., evenings or weekends) for medical advice. True emergencies went to the Emergency Department, and others knew we could see them at their convenience the next day.

The other big "ah-ha" was the difference in productivity between two physicians with similar patients and the same EMR within the same office. Within 1 month of implementing our EMR, I was typically finished with all documentation for my 28–35 patients that day and out the back door about the same time that the final patient was checking out with the receptionist. The net result was that I shaved about 2–3 h off my daily office schedule. Prior to the EMR, I would often go home with a stack of charts that I would dictate that evening, since I invariably did not do my dictations real time. Once the EMR was live, I found that I would take my history, do my exam, then document while the patient was in the room. I frequently found that I had additional questions I could then ask of the patient. My documentation became better since I was no longer trying to recall the patient from among a day's work while dictating in the evening. In addition, I took the time to note a more personal item in each record that would better connect me to the patient at a future visit. I would say, "Mrs. Jones, how is your niece doing in her first year at Harvard?" Typically, she would reply, "Oh, Dr. Smith, how do you keep track of all these things?"

I would also personally demonstrate to patients how the computer would perform drug–drug and drug–allergy interactions on new prescriptions, as well as producing a variety of patient education leaflets. By involving the patients, they soon saw that the EMR as a benefit, and not an intruder, into the patient–physician relationship. Yet even today I see physicians and nurses complaining about the EMR in front of patients, rather than promoting the opportunities the EMR affords to medical decision making and patient care.

In 1994–1995, I had my first opportunity in hospital clinical systems implementation through chairing the physician informatics committee at our local HCA (Hospital Corporation of America) as we deployed Meditech's clinical system throughout the ten hospitals of Tampa Bay. I found the experience energizing and saw a bigger picture as we were able to share secure patient information across hospitals and well as remotely access the system from the office. That year I became a 2-year transition from practicing medicine.

During 1999 through the first half of 2001, my friend Martice Nicks and I spent much of our waking hours developing business process models of how health information and data currently flowed and could flow if the industry was committed to unify under a seamless information management model. Our company, Cognitive Analysis, Inc. (CAI), brought together people from different disciplines to look at transforming health information management. Martice, coming from nuclear environmental engineering, and I, from healthcare, shared a common vision of tackling this fragmented cottage industry. We recognized the complexity of the healthcare industry and began to apply concepts that the nuclear power industry had leveraged following the Chernobyl and Three Mile Island accidents. We found encouragement in the Institute of Medicine's *To Err is Human…*[4] report in November 1999 and in the Business Roundtable's formation of the Leapfrog Group.[5] However, running low on cash, and venture capital gone due to the "dot.com" bubble bursting, we dissolved CAI in mid-2001 and I went to work for Cerner Corporation, as a physician executive on the Care Transformation Team.

While at Cerner, I had the opportunity to first identify ways to optimize existing clinical information installations, while having a hand in early adoption of CPOE on a commercial platform. Not only did Cerner leadership have a great vision for the future, but the drive and dedication of associates was endless. Cerner has a great culture of innovation and collaboration and the Care Transformation Team was at the forefront of optimization and change management.

In 2003, I transitioned as a physician in consulting at Cerner Corporation into a dual role at the Adventist Health System (AHS). I became the Vice President of

---

[4] IOM. To err is human: building a safer health system. Institute of Medicine Report. 1999.

[5] Leapfrog Group for Patient Safety at www.leapfroggroup.org.

Medical Affairs at the East Pasco Medical Center (now Florida Hospital Zephyrhills) in Zephyrhills, Florida. Simultaneously I would contribute my knowledge at the corporate level as the Chief Medical Information Officer (CMIO). I had previously consulted with AHS in my role at Cerner and befriended its Chief Medical Officer, Dr. Loran Hauck, an industry pioneer, who had first published positive outcomes of utilizing clinical pathways (today, evidence-based medicine) through paper-based order sets,[6] another of those giants in the industry. I also had the blessing to report to Brent Snyder, senior finance officer and chief information officer, for AHS and another true believer in cutting-edge clinical information systems.

The second blessing came in March 2005 when we were ready to launch our first CPOE site in May. We found that there was a possibility that another health system would acquire the pilot hospital by end of year. Knowing how these things work, it seemed unreasonable to bring up a medical staff on CPOE knowing that there was a high likelihood that their new owner would rip out their CPOE system and replace it with a standard EMR (electronic medical record), since most health systems were not ready to embrace CPOE in 2005.

Some very special experiences came from that ordeal, however. First, I realized that the whole concept of an admission order set was flawed. My experience to that time was in making "soup to nuts" order sets that included everything you needed to admit a patient with a condition such as pneumonia or heart failure. The "ah-ha" however was patients today almost all have comorbidities, such as the patient with pneumonia, worsening his heart failure and his diabetes. In the paper world, we just ignored duplicate orders. However, in the electronic CPOE world, this creates endless reconciliation of duplicates by the ordering physician. There had to be a better way. Therefore, we developed our "plug and play" model (see Chap. 2) that other health systems would adopt, and we still use today.

We also realized that we would need to create a sustainable model to produce large-scale order set content and maintain it across 37 hospitals (soon to be 44 hospitals). We wanted a reproducible model that we could highly leverage. We will discuss that topic further in Chap. 2.

Therefore, we proceeded to install our EMR model, minus CPOE, through January of 2008 to 25 hospitals in a very rapid, "big bang" fashion, and put CPOE on the back burner for the next 2 years. In addition, I left my dual role and became a full-time CMIO in August 2007 to focus on CPOE planning. This gave us late 2007 and all of 2008 to plan for two house-wide hospital pilots in early 2009. What I had gained, though, as a VP at Florida Hospital Zephyrhills was an appreciation of the culture, climate, and operations of a community hospital within AHS. This knowledge proved very useful in planning a large-scale, rapid rollout of CPOE across 26 hospitals in nine states. Moreover, if you were counting, you saw we started with 25 hospitals and ended with implementing 26. In addition, we have five new (four through merger/acquisition) hospitals on tap for 2012. We will automate

---

[6] Hauck LD, Adler LM, Mulla ZD. Clinical pathway care improves outcomes among patients hospitalized for community-acquired pneumonia. Ann Epidemiol. 2004;14:669–75.

them with our full suite of revenue cycle and clinical systems, including CPOE, physician documentation, and bar-code medication scanning.

In this book, I will share CPOE experiences, and then point out some key principles and lessons learned along the way; not only from the AHS project but also from other CPOE projects in my career. My hope is that you will read the book once, and then refer often to the different chapters to deal with opportunities that will help you right now with a current project and provide some thoughts for your future project. In addition, each chapter concludes with a "fingernails on the chalkboard" section of warning signs that you should heed. I hope that these will provide some reality and humor during this process.

As we journey together, I will be introducing you to a variety of books and resources that will help you find your way. I can only hope that you find this book useful to you, your team, and to your many future successes. Moreover, I look forward to your comments and thoughts on the topic via email: phil@medmorph. com.

August 2, 2011

Acknowledgments

I would like to thank the countless people who have contributed to my journey in healthcare informatics, leading to this book. At my current role at the Adventist Health System, I must first thank Loran Hauck, SVP and Chief Medical Officer, who has been my partner and friend throughout the CPOE process at AHS. Loran is not only a pioneer in demonstrating the benefits of evidence-based medicine in the hospital setting, but leads the Office of Clinical Effectiveness, who developed and now maintains all the AHS CPOE content. I also thank Loran for being the first to read this manuscript and provide feedback to the process.

Brent Snyder and John McLendon, both as CIOs at the Adventist Health System (AHS), who have mentored and encouraged both my development and innovation as well as supporting this effort of sharing our CPOE experiences to the world. John's belief in this project was been encouraging. Brent took the time to also review the manuscript and help me sharpen it in places. Both of these men are true leaders in IT.

In addition, I must thank Dr. Don Jernigan, CEO, and Terry Shaw, CFO/COO, of Adventist Health System, who, with Brent, have provided the vision and resources to drive adoption of clinical information systems across the enterprise. I also thank Melanie Lawhorn, in our Communications Office, who has encouraged my writing as editor for my internal blogs, and assisted me through countless hours of media interviews.

Jackie Willis, VP and CCIO (Chief Clinical Information Officer), and Judy Best, VP of business systems at Adventist Health Information Systems (AHS-IS), who work tirelessly with our teams to constantly improve our systems and keep them running.

From our teams at AHS, Charol Martindale has allowed me to use her two hopes and one fear exercise to share with the reader. This filled a need to replace an exercise that I had previously used at earlier implementations. Charol's idea proved to be a great ice-breaker for our executive workshops. Heather Linn has repeatedly provided some of the common phrases and "fingernails on the chalkboard" regarding change management. In addition, Judi Reed helped me to refine my thoughts on how best to support those folk, who every day support our doctors, with CPOE.

Moreover, our medical directors, Drs. Kshitij "Tij" Saxena, Raj Gopalan, Qammer Bokhari, and Michael Wiederhold, have brought their own strengths and energies to lead CPOE efforts and help to refine the physician roles for CPOE projects. Methodologies become stronger as men as these have led our physician engagement efforts. They have been excellent students of the methodologies of this book, and have applied it with their own successes. They have helped me focus the roles and responsibilities of physician champions in Chap. 5.

In addition, there have been the teams of people, at AHS as well as Cerner Corporation, who have contributed to the solid nature of CPOE and have helped me to refine further, the methodologies and results. You know who you are, and I thank you.

My special thanks to Izzy Justice, who was my first hands-on mentor in change management, and John Kotter, whom I am yet to meet, and yet has influenced me greatly through his numerous publications and his book, *Leading Change*. In addition, I must acknowledge Dana Alexander, who first applied the above change management concepts and tools with me for a major CPOE project. She also introduced me to the *Denison Organizational Culture Survey*, which has proved to be a valuable tool in our CPOE readiness assessment process.

I thank Ari Black and Dan Denison at Denison Consulting for providing graphics for Chap. 6. Dan's company is a fantastic resource for any industry that must embrace change.

Thanks to Neal Patterson, CEO of Cerner Corporation, for sharing his ever-growing vision for the healthcare industry, and Paul Gorup, co-founder, who has always been there with the actual resources to support innovations. They have committed resources to improve clinical decision support (CDS), a powerful foundation for anyone wanting to realize benefits and patient safety from CPOE.

Over the past 12 years, there have been phenomenal CEOs and executive teams who have demonstrated great faith in committing to the change management methodology for these CPOE projects. Thanks for the belief and helping to make it better. My personal apologies for all the lessons-learned we experienced through the last 12 years.

I must acknowledge the countless others, such as project managers, informatics, IT leads, trainers, physician support liaisons, hospital employees, and medical staffs, who have embraced CPOE and continue to help optimize the process. You have indirectly helped develop the book as you successfully managed change and implemented CPOE across North America.

I must acknowledge Scott Pitman, my first CEO at AHS, who taught me the importance of "shields and phasers" in protecting a team who are taking risks and doing great things. Thanks for being a shield and helping to improve my phasers. The reader will understand this later in the book.

In addition, I offer thanks to Drs. Jeff Rose, Dick Tayrien, J. Michael Kramer, and Scott Weingarten. They have worked with Loran and me to found the Care Collaborative, leveraging the experience of four large U.S. health systems and Zynx Health in producing new CPOE content for community hospitals. Organizations that have the opportunity to work with any of these physicians are truly blessed.

Jeff was also my boss at Cerner Corporation and first introduced me to *Leading Change* (Kotter, 1996), a pivotal book in my development of CPOE methodologies. Jeff, I was paying attention!

I thank my family: Beth, my wife, for supporting my crazy work schedule through the years and time to write this book while maintaining a huge project schedule; Amy Jensen, my daughter, for repeatedly reviewing and editing the original book proposal and manuscript, and her husband Van Jensen, himself a published author, for his encouragement and advice throughout the process.

I cannot express my pleasure enough, that Dr. Bill Bria, co-founder of AMDIS (Association of Medical Directors of Information Systems), took time to review the manuscript and write his foreword to the book. Bill, you are a true leader of leaders in this industry, and I thank you dearly for taking the time to read the manuscript and offer your encouragement through the process.

Finally, I offer my sincere thanks and appreciation to Grant Weston, my editor, at Springer, for championing the book proposal and leading me through the process.

Contents

Chapter 1
Why the Concern for CPOE

Abstract This chapter briefly covers the origin of Computerized Provider Order Entry (CPOE) and how the 2009 American Recovery and Reinvestment Act (also known as the US Stimulus bill) provided funds to acceleration CPOE adoption. The author introduces Four Principles to guide clinical IT (information technology) projects.

> The more things change, the more they stay the same
>
> – Jean-Baptiste Alphonse Karr (translated from French)

In June of 1973, a group of pioneers from Lockheed-Martin brought a new clinical computer system live at El Camino Hospital in Mountain View, California. This system would replace the doctors' handwritten orders with orders entered directly into a computer the birth of what the industry would later call computerized provider order entry or CPOE. By 2008, about 10 % of U.S. hospitals had adopted computerized provider order entry,[1] and systems now include not only ordering, but also the inclusion of clinical decision support (CDS). Based on other technology adoptions[2] like radio, television and personal computers, one might predict that it would take another 35 years for 90 % of hospitals to adopt CPOE. Despite 92 % of the published articles on CPOE touting benefits to patient safety, quality and outcomes,[3] CPOE adoption was still creeping along with only a few hospitals activating full CPOE annually. In addition, Rand Corporation published a study in 2005 on the potential reduction of costs through wide adoption of healthcare IT.[4] CPOE and EHR adoption needed a catalyst.

---

[1] Though the original name for CPOE was computerized physician order entry, today most refer to computerized provider or prescriber order entry to acknowledge mid-lever providers/prescribers such as physician assistants and advanced practice nurses.

[2] Dent HS Jr. The roaring 2000s: building the wealth and life style you desire in the greatest boom in history. New York: Simon and Schuster; 1998.

[3] Buntin MB, Burke MF, Hoaglin MC, Blumenthal D. The benefits of health information technology. A review of the recent literature shows predominantly positive results. Health Aff. 2011;30:3, 464–71.

[4] Girosi F, Meili RC, Scoville R. Extrapolating evidence of health information technology savings and costs. Santa Monica: RAND Corporation; 2005. http://www.rand.org/pubs/monographs/MG410.

P.A. Smith, *Making Computerized Provider Order Entry Work*,
Health Information Technology Standards,
DOI 10.1007/978-1-4471-4243-0_1, © Springer-Verlag London 2013

With the stroke of the pen in February 2009, United States President Barack Obama signed into law the $800 billion American Recovery and Reinvestment Act of 2009 (ARRA)[5] While the "stimulus bill" had numerous provisions for federal investment in infrastructure projects, it also represented a huge commitment to healthcare information technology (HIT) under the section now known as ARRA HITECH. With billions of dollars of federal incentives available, hospitals and physicians are attempting to demonstrate "meaningful use of certified EHR technology." This has become the burning platform needed by many hospitals and physician offices to pursue CPOE and other aspects of electronic health records.

While ARRA HITECH is also providing grants for new clinical IT training programs, industry leaders report that there is currently a deficit of trained clinicians capable of implementing these new initiatives. In addition to CPOE, HITECH will push automation of clinical outcomes, electronic physician documentation, e-Prescribing, and Health Information Exchanges (HIE).

As too few experienced persons pursue too many projects, the industry may see an increase in project failures, which will send ripples throughout healthcare IT, leading to confusion, pushback, or even slowing/cancellation of major projects. This book may provide some ideas that can help professionals think through the steps toward project success.

1.1 Four Principles

As I have worked with physicians on large, complex health care projects these past 20 years, I have devised four principles that have consistently guided successful projects. Let me explain each of them:

1. Every day, every person in health care comes to work planning to do their best for the patients.
2. Every day, every person in health care comes to work listening to the same radio station, WII-FM ("What's in it for me?").
3. Automating broken processes gets you to the wrong place quicker.
4. Today's problems were yesterday's solutions.

These four principles have been both a barometer and a checklist for me over the past two decades. Taken together, these principles can keep you on track as you navigate the dangerous waters of major projects from design, activation and adoption. So let us take them one at a time and better understand what they mean. Then we can apply them throughout the book as we tackle the major steps to project success.

Every day, every person in health care comes to work planning to do their best for the patients.

People get into healthcare because they have a passion to make a difference. This is the principle of "higher calling". Almost every doctor, nurse, therapist, technician

---

[5] For more information on ARRA, visit www.hhs.gov/recovery.

or any other healthcare worker strive to make a difference in the lives of their patients. You see it in their commitment, in their faces and in their work ethic. They study hard, they work hard, and they understand the high stakes of dealing with life and death issues. No one comes to work wanting to commit an error, omit some treatment, or to do less than his/her personal best. Yet each human being is capable of making an error, even on a good day. Fortunately, harm rarely occurs from a single person making a single error.

Most harm, in our experience, occurs when a cascade of errors occurs, processes are lax, and/or end-users do not follow recommended procedures. Health care has made great strides in the past 20 years to create better systems, to simplify processes, and to provide error trapping (e.g., alerts and clinical decision support). One thing is clear: people in healthcare suffer a personal, emotional cost whenever an error occurs, especially if patient harm is the result. The person who does set out to do harm, is a very rare exception to the norm. From this principle arises two important points: (1) Don't ever communicate that you are engineering a new process to make it "idiot-proof", and (2) While patient safety and great outcomes are important to everyone in healthcare, principle #2 below often trumps this principle.

People do not make mistakes because they are idiots. They make mistakes because we are human, and because our systems have not yet matured to accommodate the natural course of human behavior. So communicating "idiot-proof" solutions only implies contempt for the basic truth of this principle. Any person thinking he/she can design and implement idiot-proof solutions probably has not been doing it for very long. In fact, the story below illustrates that you can never predict what others are thinking.

> I learned very early in my career that physicians often believe that what they have been doing since medical school and residency always represents the best practice. When new evidence recommends that we change the techniques or medications that we use, many physicians have a natural resistance to change. On more than one occasion, I have had a physician, in a defensive tone, reply, "You mean you are telling me that I've been doing it wrong all these years?" Now that same physician is probably performing laparoscopic surgery for a procedure that he learned to do by open incision, but he misses that connection in his defensiveness.
>
> At that moment, we must overcome the defensiveness and process the evidence openly. As the physician calms down and begins to consider the evidence, he/she begins to acknowledge the patient safety aspect and becomes more open to discussion. By having patient safety as our ultimate outcome, the project team is able to move CPOE forward with less resistance.

While patient safety and great outcomes are always an overall objective, there are frequently distractions that seem to get in the way. Principle #2 explains the phenomenon.

Every day, every person in health care comes to work listening to the same radio station, WII-FM.

WII-FM of course is the abbreviation for "What's in it for me?" While everyone in health care is passionate and committed to a good patient outcome, it is important to realize that every new advancement and process must add some personal benefit to the person expected to adopt it. Typically, a person will take the "path of least resistance" in his/her day, unless some new process can add some personal value. For physicians, that value typically comes as more time, more money or more peace of mind. In addition, unless we internalize the value of a new process or procedure, we will fall back to our old ways with resistance, work-a-rounds, or even outright rebellion. As we adopt new processes and new technologies, it is critical we clearly communicate what the benefit will be to the individual who must make the change. This might include a more efficient process, new cues, less effort, or incentives, to name a few. Of course, each person in health care comes to work with principle #1. However, it is principle #2 that smoothes adoption and creates lasting change. You may refer to Principle #2 as the "law of self-interest".

I encountered a hospital recently where the main CPOE message was, "We are doing CPOE to collect the Meaningful Use dollars." The doctors were upset that the hospital was disrupting their daily work patterns to collect "millions of dollars, while they are turning us into secretaries." Once this becomes the stated driver for CPOE, you experience more resistance from the medical staff, and ultimately the staff follows suit.

Failing to find and state value for your doctors and nurses is lazy and creates "ill-will" that takes much effort to overcome. Physicians realize that CPOE is hard and will take much effort on everyone's part to be successful. However, they also need to hear from leadership the direct value to the physician from CPOE. Just like the hospital expects a return on investment from CPOE, the medical staff looks for time, money or peace of mind. You should have a clear value in mind for each of your major stakeholder groups, especially your physicians.

Automating broken processes gets you to the wrong place quicker
Many think that new technology is often the solution to things that are no longer working in an organization. Take automating clinical processes as an example. Many clinical processes are inherently inefficient and needlessly complex. Often there is no acknowledgement of this because the process crosses the paths on many different individuals in many different locations or departments. In fact, flowcharting the process often reveals issues that have persisted for years. Often, the person in the midst of the complex process knows primarily what they do, and a little bit about what the people immediately before and immediately after them do in the process. Yet there may be five or more hand-offs before the process is completed.

The workflow team in the Emergency Department (ED) at one pre-CPOE hospital identified a process that involved the registration clerk photocopying the visit encounter notes following every ED visit, stapling them together and putting them in an "out basket." No one knew why the copying was necessary; they had repeated this ritual for several years. A volunteer would pick up these copies and hand-carry them across the hospital and deposit them into an "in basket" in the Pharmacy. Once the pharmacist got to the "in basket", he would drop the encounter record into the shredder bin for destruction. When our analyst asked why this process was occurring, the pharmacist replied, "We had reviewed all the ED records manually in the past, but now do this electronically in the EHR. We have told the ED to quit sending these up, but they continue to send them anyway." The hospital CEO stopped this unnecessary process that day, well in advance of CPOE and immediately challenged his team to identify other examples of waste or duplication. All of us are familiar with the old adage, "That's just the way we have always done it around here."

Another error is not thinking through how to leverage automation to eliminate unnecessary or inefficient steps in the process – automating the paper processes as a result. Using lean techniques, designers can often eliminate several steps and remove sub-processes that are "non-value" added. As the designer provides "transparency" around the process, the end-users can begin to identify opportunities to streamline workflow and minimize wasted steps. It is critical that the design engage the actual end-users in this stage of the process. The designer should document decisions and frequently asked questions as well as identify the value statements important to the end-users. The project team then leverages this information to achieve buy-in and adoption of the new processes.

An example of this at AHS was the discharge process. Prior to CPOE, a doctor would tell the patient that he/she would be "discharging them that day and please have your family come in to take you home." Prior to CPOE, however, the nurses reported that it would take about 4–6 h to gather all the information together and complete the discharge. This would greatly frustrate the family member who took off work, only to sit for several hours waiting. As discussed later in the book, the team at AHS redesigned the CPOE discharge process. As a result, the patient typically left the hospital within 30 min of the doctor writing the discharge order. The patients, nurses and doctors have all seen this as a benefit of the new process. However, some units have held on to their old discharge process and not seen this benefit.

Commonly, the team's initial efforts of automation may result in flaws or miss sub-processes and situations (i.e. "use-cases") that they did not plan or consider. Fortunately, the end-users tend to identify many of these during training or during the first 30 days post implementation. The design team may experience embarrassment at this result; however, a mature team will see this as an opportunity. The team humbly can address the deficiencies and thoughtfully work through these sub-processes and determine a solution to validate. While the first attempt may not be the final solution, it allows the team to work together and builds confidence and assurance that no matters what happens, the team will address and overcome the immediate challenges.

In addition, this principle reminds us that we must properly manage expectations for the project. The phrase, "under promise and over deliver" helps us to keep the proper perspective as we communicate to the end-users as well as to the facility leadership. This is the "law of managing expectations."

Moreover, CPOE implementation may expose areas in which the hospital may improve accountability. The largest area, in our experience, has been in clearly defining the difference between clinical processes and medical decision-making. The author will address that in more detail in a later chapter.

Today's problems were yesterday's solutions.

I started using this phrase over 30 years ago while in college and it has always kept me humble (I honestly do not know if I coined it or heard it back then.). While principle #3 deals with immediate cause and effect, principle #4 deals with long-term consequences. It is important to recognize that in one's efforts to fix some obvious issue or problem, a new (not so obvious) problem often results down the road, and a more complex one at that. As Einstein said, "We cannot solve our problems with the same thinking we used when we created them." Always recognize that in the rush to solve problems, one may create unintended consequences, which may not even be apparent for some time. Therefore, look for iterative solutions to complex problems. Do not expect solutions to come easy or be simple. Moreover, do not expect to have all the answers up front. Do your initial analysis, move forward cautiously, then identify where sequential adaptations and improvements (enhancements) need to occur. Two points of danger occur: analysis paralysis, in which you never move forward until you have everything perfectly figured out; and foolhardy implementation, rushing in with your "perfect" solution, only to find that you are in over your head with an unworkable solution. This is the "law of unintended consequences."

> Most of us in clinical IT have seen this play out in the area of "hard-stops" in the EHR. The concept is that you engineer some required documentation that must occur in the workflow in order for the nurse or physician to proceed to the next step. These rarely work out, since for every "rule" in healthcare, we eventually find an "exception." In addition, the exception may be in midst of the physician/ nurse providing some life-saving care. Typically, we design alerts or "soft-stops" for these scenarios. We provide some type of warning to alert the user, but then give them the option to proceed, with or without some reason for overriding.

CPOE, itself, presents some new "unintended consequences." One may design a system to promote safety, and inadvertently drive their end-users to select the wrong meds, wrong doses or wrong routes of administration. For more on this topic, one should familiarize himself with the work of the Physician Order Entry Team (POET) at the Oregon Health and Science University.[6]

To apply these four principles, one should look at current or past project challenges to examine how a team might gain insights from them. From the analysis, the team may find new opportunities for discussion that may prove helpful. Then, the team will be able to utilize them to anticipate issues or proactively prevent problems during future projects.

Moreover, the hospital of the twenty-first century should focus on three core competences: healthcare delivery, information management, and sound financial management. CPOE provides a wealth of data and information that help hospitals to achieve improved clinical, operational and financial outcomes. Hospital executives

---

[6] This excellent resource is at www.cpoe.org. This site presents the results of research by the Physician Order Entry Team (POET) at Oregon Health & Science University.

should view CPOE as a strategic initiative. As they access better real-time data, they can make more-informed decisions in these areas and make early course directions when they do not achieve the results they expected. The author will discuss this further in later chapters.

1.2   Key Points

- ARRA HITECH has become a catalyst for EHR/CPOE adoption
- Assume healthcare workers have a high-calling for patient care
- Assume everyone responds to self-interest
- Automating broken processes will get you the wrong result quicker
- New solutions will generate new problems down the road

1.3   Fingernails on the Chalkboard

My "red flags" on these topics occur with the following comments/observations:

- **"Let's do CPOE this year so that we can collect the Meaningful Use dollars!"**
  Your employees and doctors do not see value in disrupting their days and workflow so that the hospital can collect a government incentive. In fact, this can often become the motto of resistance for a CPOE project as physicians claim that you are only doing CPOE for the money. Your strong vision for the project also needs to generate value to your stakeholders, namely your Board, your employees and your medical staff.
- **"We are putting in the new EHR to catch all the mistakes our doctors/nurses are making**."
  Doctors and nurses feel great about the care they delivery and become defensive when you make such comments. Yet we all know the even on our best days, we all overlook information and make less than optimal decisions. It is critical to come to your team with specific data on where opportunities exist and how we plan to improve our patient care processes. Armed with data, your team will see opportunities to improve the patient care process through your CPOE project.
- **"Get on board with the project, or you will be looking for a new job."**
  No one gets excited about a project that begins with threats. Sell the value to your team up front and they will come along with you. This is important with positions, such as unit clerks/secretaries (noted below), who will experience a major change in their daily activities once you implement CPOE.
- **"We are doing this to cut costs for the hospital"**
  While everyone supports cutting costs, that often means cutting jobs. You can make a case for helping everyone be more productive and efficient through new processes as we free up bandwidth and resources.

- **"We are doing CPOE to eliminate the unit clerks."**
  Unit clerks have the ear of both the nurses and the doctors. They will derail a CPOE project if they believe that you are trying to eliminate their job. Instead, you must actively engage them early and help them understand the opportunities they will have as you bring CPOE live. There will be more on this topic in Chap. 5.
- **"Our nurses/doctors don't have the time to participate in design sessions."**
  It is sometimes a challenge to engage doctors and nurses, and it ensures a disaster if you do not engage them. We will discuss this in depth in chapter 7.
- **"Just figure it out, and we will make the nurses follow the new processes!"**
  Part of the success of CPOE is designing leaner processes that create new efficiencies and improved patient care. When the front-line nurses get involved in designing the new workflows, they will be more likely to actually follow them, rather than work around them. You will avoid implementation rebellion when nurses have "skin in the game" up front.
- **"Let's not worry about that now, since CPOE will solve that problem."**
  You can leverage your CPOE project as a great opportunity to better understand your current inefficiencies and design a better workflow(s) that you can implement either before, with, or after CPOE activation. Rarely does CPOE fix problems that existed unless you give them special attention in the process. Typically, you will accelerate problems once CPOE goes live.
- **When you see a lack of committed resources to train new employees/doctors and ensure ongoing competencies of end-users**.
  As you go live with CPOE, it is a 1-day event. The real work is in stabilizing your new system and then finding opportunities to optimize your processes. Therefore, you must keep your training materials and trainers up to date on these new processes. As new doctors and employees enter the system, you must train them on how you do business today, and not on what you were teaching when you first brought your system live. Otherwise, you will be discouraging your newest users and losing the benefit of your optimization processes.
- **Beware, if you have no plan for optimization of processes following implementation and stabilization**.
  The end-users using your EHR are your best sources of understanding where you must focus your efforts to achieve improved clinical, financial and operational outcomes. Often, post activation, the design and implementation teams are already working on subsequent projects or not involved in seeing how your end-users are using the EHR/CPOE. If you fail to staff your optimization efforts, you are failing to reap the full benefits of your automation efforts.
- **Plan to fail if you do not have doctors contributing to your project**.
  Though most doctors will choose not to participate on your project, you will need physicians who will commit time for review and feedback during several key points in the process.

Chapter 2
Vision: How You Start

Abstract This chapter explains the importance of vision for successful CPOE projects. The author provides a structure for developing and managing order set content for a CPOE project. In addition, he discusses how to one plans the initial scope of their CPOE project. The author stresses that patient safety is the best reason for a hospital or health system to pursue a CPOE project.

> *Where there is no vision, the people perish:*
> *– Proverbs 29:18 (Bible, King James Version)*

Why start with vision? Because if you do not get vision right, you are doomed to failure. Whether you are tackling CPOE or any other large-scale initiative, vision is what determines what you are actually trying to accomplish and why.

Over the years, I had multiple opportunities to assess projects that had failed, were failing, or seriously stalled. Each time, I have observed a lack of clear vision from the senior leadership. Typically, the IT department has an idea why the project is proceeding, but not the CEO and senior executives. The worst case occurred in the early 2000s, when the senior executives, 1 month prior to CPOE activation, did not even know that CPOE meant that physicians would be entering orders into the computer and no longer writing them. It was news to their medical staff as well. Yet the project team had built the platform and was ready to execute! I was unpopular when I recommended that they were months away from being able to activate CPOE. Fortunately, the CEO did get involved and many months later saw a very successful implementation.

At the Adventist Health System (AHS), "Deploying clinical information systems and having CPOE well under way" was the leading statement for the 2010 Vision Statement. The senior leadership made it clear from the beginning that our EHR and CPOE were corporate initiatives and not just IT initiatives. This visibility places it in the annual report, before the Board, and at the front and center of strategic discussions. Senior leadership determines whether CPOE is the highest priority, or just another project only affecting a small group within the system.

Why is this important in the case of CPOE? First, CPOE affects almost every workflow in the hospital. Therefore, it requires every department and unit of the hospital to understand how CPOE affects them and how to leverage it for improved efficiency. In addition, CPOE changes the physician's workflow from one

P.A. Smith, *Making Computerized Provider Order Entry Work*,
Health Information Technology Standards,
DOI 10.1007/978-1-4471-4243-0_2, © Springer-Verlag London 2013

of viewing information and handwriting orders to total interaction with the EHR. Handwritten orders have been the norm for years, so having the doctors perform computerized order entry is a major change for their workflow. Moreover, each CEO, in the community hospital, has physician satisfaction as a core responsibility. The hospital does not employ these physicians or award academic appointments. The CEO and medical staff form a relationship that depends on mutual trust and benefit. Therefore, getting physicians on board and participating with this change is critical. The CEO does not want, and cannot afford, to alienate the medical staff in the process.

Coupled with the Vision Statement, AHS clearly identified CPOE as an opportunity to improve patient safety while creating a consistent platform to deliver clinical best practices and evidence-based medicine recommendations to the end-users. This conclusion came after 10 years of medical staffs utilizing these pathways as paper-based order sets on only about 40 % of qualifying patients. The ultimate vision has always been to "hard-wire" evidence-based medicine into the physician's "path-of-least-resistance" workflow.

After the first two pilot hospitals went live with CPOE, Don Jernigan, the AHS chief executive officer (CEO), validated the vision through strong messages to the hospital CEOs at the annual meeting, saying, "Seeing CPOE go live at these two hospitals represented some of the proudest moments of my career." Dr. Jernigan's message, coupled with the 2010 Vision Statement, created a clear mandate to the CEOs and their hospitals that would follow the pilots. One cannot put a price tag on your CEOs public support.

Once you cast your vision, then all the fun work begins. What will the project encompass (i.e. What is the scope)? What is the roadmap? How do we begin? How will we make decisions? You will find detailed answers to these important questions in the subsequent chapters. I always like to start with Stephen R. Covey's[1] analogy of filling a bucket with rocks, gravel, sand and water – always start with the "big rocks" first.

2.1 Building Up from the Vision

The "big rocks" for AHS were how to achieve the vision of "hard-wiring" evidence-based medicine and promote patient safety. While the author had seen other health systems and hospitals use other approaches, it was obvious how to set up the program at AHS.

From the evidence-based medicine aspect, it became clear that while there are regional differences in how our hospitals operate and in the level of resources available (i.e., local variation), AHS wanted to fully leverage clinical guidelines and best practice for diseases and conditions for which evidence exists. For example, the American College of Cardiology regularly updates its guidelines on the treatment of

---

[1] Covey SR. The seven habits of highly effective people. New York: Fireside; 1989.

acute ST-elevated myocardial infarction[2] (acute STEMI, or heart attack). This then becomes the standard of care that we expect physicians to follow regardless of whether they practice at a large hospital in Florida or at a small critical access hospital in Wisconsin. This meant a move from "experience-based medicine" in which decisions on order set content for acute STEMI rests in the hands of the local medical staff, to a more universal approach, of deploying a common "evidence-based" order set at a corporate level, that would be shared by all. The common phrase by AHS Chief Medical Officer Dr. Loran Hauck became "we are not advocating a standardized approach to the practice of medicine by our physician, but rather that they practice to a standard." This was a change in approach to the paper order set days, when the Office of Medical Affairs sent an Acute STEMI template to each hospital for local revisions and printing, to a common electronic order set shared by all AHS hospitals.

The challenge then was to solve two issues. How does one provide the infrastructure to keep corporate content up to date, and how does one deal with the difference in resources available to hospitals of varying sizes, structure and markets? Fortunately, the Chief Medical Officer had recently expanded his department from an Office of Medical Affairs, into the AHS Office of Clinical Effectiveness (OCE). This proved a timely change that helped to drive the solution to our infrastructure issue.

2.2 Managing Order Set Content

AHS tackled content first, since they already had a Corporate Physician Committee (CPC) to review and develop evidence-based content and a relationship with Zynx Health,[3] a provider of evidence-based content. However, we knew the volunteer army of community physicians, nurses and clinical pharmacists could not manage the volume of content needed to implement CPOE. Previously, the CPC had developed and maintained content on about ten conditions, diseases, and operations through monthly meetings and a few workgroups. In assessing what they needed, they looked at all discharge diagnoses for the prior 2 years and determined what represented the top 85 % of conditions/diseases that they were managing in the hospitals. In addition, they identified 64 common presentations of signs and symptoms for the Emergency Department and several dozen protocols such as anticoagulation management. All told, this represented a need for about 550 order sets to have a robust catalogue. The principle for these order sets was that they were universal and the hospitals would not modify locally. As a comparison, the author has done CPOE projects with as few as 35 order sets and as many as 2,000.

---

[2] ACC/AHA. ACC/AHA guidelines for the management of patients with ST-elevation myocardial infarction. J Am Coll Cardiol. 2004;44:671–719.

[3] www.ZynxHealth.com.

For admitting patients to the hospitals, AHS realized the hospitals varied in size, structure and resources, so committed to build a localized admission order set for each type of unit by hospital. The team called these order sets "Admit to Venue", and named them for the unit to which they applied. So in the case of Florida Hospital Zephyrhills (FHZ), the Admit to Venues included:

- Admit to Med/Surg/Telemetry FHZ
- Admit to ICU FHZ
- Admit to Labor FHZ
- Admit to Peds FHZ
- Admit to Behavioral Health FHZ

To promote local collaboration on the Admit to Venue design, the hospital's Medical Executive Committee, which governs the Medical Staff, became the approving group of the content for the local Admit to Venues. The OCE team would serve as content editors, to ensure that identified outmoded practices did not make it into these order sets.

Knowing that the content would have to be solid for over 9,000 community physicians to accept, they decided that the OCE would be the owner of all corporate order set content. This proved to be a wise decision.

In previous CPOE projects, a physician associated with the IT team, such as the CMIO or a medical director, would own content for all order sets. They would then have endless meetings with physicians by specialty and try to iron out the best order set to meet the needs of that group. While the author has observed some skilled physician consultants in my career facilitate these "rapid order set design sessions," the more likely result is that these sessions derail from local politics and opinions. Typically, one or two outspoken physicians will dominate the session with his/her "expert opinion" often overriding even the strongest evidence, and shut down all other collaboration. An example brings clarity to this concept.

The setting was a 2-day, rapid order set design session for the Department of Orthopedics at a multi-hospital system (around 2002). The group included a couple of orthopedic surgeons, nurses, surgical technicians and unit clerks. By the second day, the group had designed three order sets, including total knee replacement, total hip replacement, and hip fracture. They were finishing up with post-operative recommendations for dosing two blood thinners, enoxaparin and warfarin, and had concluded that "mini-dose heparin" was no longer an evidence-based alternative to prevent the post-operative, life-threatening complication of blood clots (today VTE, or venous thromboembolism). As the group was ready to leave, after two hard nights of work, a lone unit clerk raised her hand and brought the process to a screeching halt, "Dr. Jones (name changed) does half the orthopedic surgery at my hospital, and he only uses mini-dose heparin on his patients."

It took about 5 min for the group to capitulate on the evidence, and agree to add mini-dose heparin to the new "evidence-based" order sets. Moreover, Dr. Jones did not even show up to participate in the process.

The physician leading content design must be a person of influence and an excellent facilitator. The result is that the process completely consumes the physician responsible for content, who then has no time left to contribute to other aspects of the project, while disenfranchising all other physicians in that specialty who are now silent. There is one principle that one should honor if you decide to pursue order set design sessions: "Always begin a design session with a draft order set for discussion. Never start with a clean slate." Through the years, the author has sat through many order set design sessions to watch a consultant start the session with a blank sheet of paper. The sessions are very painful, drawn out, and the participants rarely come to quick consensus. It is much more productive to know the evidence surrounding the topic, look at what the physicians are already doing, point out where they already agree and use the collaboration time to tackle a few areas where experience-based medicine has kept them from following the evidence. In addition, feeding doctors at these events always seems to make them work out better.

In reviewing the work ahead at AHS, they planned for OCE to hire a full time medical director over content, to work with a team of a project manager, three nurses, a part-time clinical pharmacist, and a librarian. Dr. Paul Garrett, from Florida Hospital Orlando, the flagship hospital, accepted this position. In addition, the two other physicians in OCE, Dr. Hauck and Dr. Doug Bechard, chief quality officer, would round out the corporate infrastructure. Overall, ten content committees were formed in the process to include practicing community physicians with subject matter expertise. These included:

- Emergency Department
- Pediatrics
- Neonatology
- Anesthesiology
- Surgery and Orthopedics
- Neurology and Neurosurgery
- Gastroenterology
- Internal Medicine and Interventional Radiology
- Psychiatry
- Cardiology and Cardiovascular Surgery

Initially AHS contracted and paid for the community physicians' time on these committees as they developed initial content. Today, most have continued to serve as volunteers. Through the years, the author has seen similar structures with more committees at academic centers and pediatric hospitals. Community hospitals may only need Medicine, Surgery, Emergency Department and Obstetrics. The important point is to have a structure, not only for order set creation, but also for the physicians' ongoing review and maintenance of the content.

Each AHS committee reviews their content at a minimum of biannually, and whenever new clinical guidelines appear. The most active has been cardiology, with major revisions at least every year. Within the CPOE electronic order sets, physicians have an active email link in which to submit immediate feedback or questions on the content. These emails automatically log a change control request assigned to the OCE for review and follow up with the physician. The end-user providers have seen hundreds of changes and enhancements that have originated through this feedback loop. The owner of any CPOE content should make sure that they have a long-term plan for ongoing order set maintenance.

2.3 Plug and Play

Knowing that patients frequently arrive at the hospital with more than one disease/condition, AHS devised an approach to order set design named "plug and play." In the paper world, admission order sets for heart failure, for example, would have all the orders to register the patient, as well as to define diet, activity, code status and vital signs. This worked fine until you admitted a patient with pneumonia and heart failure. If the physician used an admission order set for heart failure along with one for pneumonia, then the unit clerk ignores the duplicates on paper as she enters these orders into the EHR. In the CPOE world, however, the ordering provider must deal with the duplicates on the front end, prior to electronic signature.

Therefore, the team determined that a provider could electronically order the Admit to Venue order set and one or more "disease/condition" order sets to cover the needs of the patient. While a change in how physicians previously ordered on paper, this proved a rapid way to enter initial orders on a patient with multiple co-morbidities, such as diabetes and heart failure in addition to pneumonia. They designated the disease/condition-specific order sets as "core content."

In addition, AHS formulated a partnership with other similar "faith-based," community health systems that were pursuing CPOE on a similar timeline and EHR. This group has since worked with Zynx Health as the Care Collaborative,[4] which now provides order set content to a significant number of hospitals in the U.S. Through this collaboration, they developed a Style Guide for the order sets to facilitate ease of communication and tested various concepts for how best to deploy the content. The most powerful achievement, however, was gathering a large number of neonatologists, neonatal nurses and advanced practice nurses to formulate a complete library of order sets for the critical care of infants in the first month of life.

The final comment on order sets for this chapter is that one must have a formal process for change control. Changes arise through factors such as evolution of EHR system design, workflow changes, new clinical guidelines, new medications or discontinued medications, new service lines, and new technologies. At AHS, the OCE works very closely with the clinical IT team to ensure that each reviews any changes prior to implementation.

---

[4] Original members of the Care Collaborative were Ascension Health, Adventist Health System, Catholic Healthcare West, Cerner Corporation, Trinity Health and Zynx Health. Today, the Care Collaborative includes Ascension Health, Adventist Health System, Catholic Healthcare West (now Dignity Health) and Zynx Health. http://www.zynxhealth.com/News/Press-Releases/2010/05/Care-Collaborative.aspx.

2.4 Visual Anchor

The visual anchor is an image that provides a clear representation of the problem. In the case of CPOE, the author likes to use two images: one of an illegible set of handwritten orders, the other the same orders clearly displayed in the EMR via CPOE. Every patient, Board member, and caregiver can relate to this image and the dangers it represents:

- Medication delays
- Medication errors
- Patient harm or even death
- Liability
- Lack of immediate clinical decision support

The image must be very strong and stand independently to represent why one is doing CPOE. While physicians and other may resist CPOE publicly and privately, it is hard for them to deny the impact of illegible orders.

To further this image, the team should have stories that relate actual benefits of CPOE orders over handwriting. At one CPOE site a physician admitted his patient to the hospital from the office, 2 days into CPOE. The story relates how she arrived at the hospital and the nurse activated her planned admission orders, only to see everyone in her care working in concert rather than in a delayed, fragmented manner. The decisive moment, however, came when the CEO asked her what she thought of her experience as one of the first CPOE admissions, and she stated, "I felt like the whole hospital was on call for me!" That story left an impression on everyone, from the patient, the caregivers, the administration, and the entire CPOE project team. The anchor gives an emotional assurance to the leadership and to the all involved. The author has included the visual anchor (Fig. 6.2) for the AHS project in Chap. 6.

2.5 Project Plan and Scope

Once executive leadership determines the vision, the project sponsor must work to define the scope of the project, begin the formal project planning, and determine resources and the timeline. It is important that the leadership of the organization translate the vision of their project into a statement of scope that allows them to achieve the vision.

The author has seen many organizations through the years fail to take the time to define a full statement of scope that will fulfill the vision. As a result, the project team may determine that CPOE, i.e. having physicians place orders electronically, defines the scope of the project. They then turn it over to a project manager, who appropriately attempts to manage the scope around merely the electronic ordering processes. Later the project predictably stalls while physician resistance increases.

The project team creatively attempts to overcome the resistance as the project manager sounds the alarm of scope creep. Moreover, if the scope of the project is too narrow at the start, then any adjustments will require the team to either extend the timeline or commit more resources.

The author recommends that you really understand the vision of the project, and that CPOE is really a process that will help you achieve your vision and goals. However, CPOE may only address the first principle in Chap. 1. Without thoughtful planning, the organization may miss the opportunity to serve the second principle as well, i.e. the "What's in it for me?" principle. The result might be that you activate CPOE, but lose sustainability as the physicians see a drop in personal productivity.

One may avoid this pitfall by considering the first two principles simultaneously. Would it not be preferable to increase patient safety and help the physicians achieve higher personal productivity? Instead of seeing CPOE as the lone goal, one should likewise seek to improve physician efficiency. While CPOE activation is a project objective, we see automating the physician workflow to achieve improved efficiency, effectiveness and patient safety as the overarching goal.[5]

Once the organization commits to the goal of automating the physicians' workflow during their CPOE process, they can begin to focus on more than just orders and the medication process. For each workflow, teams need to document the current state processes. It is important that current state documentation reflect actual workflows, and not a manager's opinion of what the processes should be. These are also great opportunities for an organization to perform pre and post-CPOE metrics. We recommend that the scope include the following processes:

- Admission processes

  - This includes admission from office to hospital, Emergency Department to hospital, post surgery to hospital, and transfer from another facility. For CPOE, we recommend that nurses own the key components of obtaining and documenting allergies, height, weight, medication history including patient compliance and last dose, and an admission assessment dataset (e.g. vital signs, history of current presentation, family and social history). The physicians should own: determination of intensity of services (e.g. critical care vs. non-critical care), admission diagnosis, admission orders, admission medication reconciliation of home (or prior venue of care) medications, and an admission History and Physical. In addition, the initial registration process becomes critical path since nurses and physicians must have an electronic encounter on which to document and order.
  - At AHS, the team noted extreme variation in the pre-CPOE metric of time between a decision to admit until nurses and doctors complete all admitting processes. They measured cycle times at each hospital and worked prior to CPOE activation to improve both quality and expediency of the nurse admission

---

[5] Amusan AA, Tongen S, Speedie SM, Mellin A. Time-saver: a time-motion study to evaluate the impact of EMR and CPOE implementation on physician efficiency. J Healthc Inf Manag. 2009;22:4.

process with tremendous improvements. One should remember Principle #3 from Sect. 1.1, and improve the process prior to CPOE. We would like to see the provider complete the orders and medication reconciliation for the CPOE admission process in 3–5 min.

- Transfer processes
  - There are several transfer processes to consider, and the components of regis- tration, nursing and provider workflows. Transfers typically include: critical care unit to non-critical care units and vice-versa, post anesthesia care to nurs- ing unit, change in attending or medical service, and transfers (i.e. discharges) to other facilities (e.g. other acute care hospitals, tertiary care hospitals, long- term acute care or rehabilitation hospitals.). Both nurses and providers should document hand-off procedures, orders reconciliation, and registration events. One would ideally like the physician to complete a transfer within the facility in 1–3 min.

- Discharge processes
  - The discharge process represents a huge opportunity for improving patient safety/satisfaction as well as nurse and physician efficiency at the time of discharge. The discharge process begins with the physician's decision to dis- charge the patient from the hospital, and includes all processes through the patient actually leaving the hospital. The author discusses this in a later chap- ter in detail. However, he has seen many CPOE projects stumble as they fail to give appropriate attention to the discharge process. The physician owns all medical decision-making steps in the process: decision to discharge, order to discharge, discharge reconciliation of medications to determine a list of home medications, diet, activity, follow-up plan for medical care and instructions regarding the primary procedure or diagnosis. All of the physician's decisions should flow seamlessly to the patient's discharge instructions in lay terminol- ogy. The physician should also review the completion of any ordered inter- ventions and comment on any exclusions for regulatory requirements (Such as why discharge plan excludes any evidence-based interventions such as daily aspirin following a heart attack). The nurse should return valuables, review the discharge plan for patient/family comprehension, educate accord- ing to the interdisciplinary plan of care, and ensure that there are no red flags such as lack of safe transport to the next venue of care or inability to under- stand the discharge instructions.
  - The discharge metrics should include current state for discharge to home, transfer to another acute care facility, transfer to other location (nursing home or assisted living facility), and in-hospital mortality (need for autopsy, release of body, and preliminary cause of death).
  - The reason for paying attention to the discharge process is that it is the last experience the patient has with the hospital and often is inefficient and inap- propriate. Many a patient has had a doctor tell him that "you can go home today," only to have their loved ones arrive at the hospital and wait 4–6 h until

the actual discharge occurs. This is mainly due to nurses trying to track down the physician to obtain all the information necessary for a safe discharge. We recommend that you take the time to design a CPOE discharge process that permits a measureable improvement in time from discharge order until the patient leaves the facility. We believe that 30 min is an average goal that one can achieve. The physician part of the discharge process, exclusive of dictating or completing a discharge summary document, should take 3–5 min on average.

- Medication reconciliation processes

  – Medication reconciliation (med rec) actually represents several sub-processes, all centered around the goal of the physician giving consideration to the patient's home medications each time a change in venue occurs. In the author's opinion, med rec is an essential process for patient safety and should be a physician responsibility for all CPOE projects.
  – Online medication reconciliation tools must be able to provide the providers with the ability to perform and reconciliation during admission, during transfers and at the time of patient discharge. The tools must permit the physician from distinguishing home medications from any inpatient medications. Admission medication reconciliation must allow the provider to continue a patient's home medications as inpatient medication orders. In addition, admission med rec should already be a physician-led process prior to CPOE. However, some facilities, in preparation for CPOE, discover that they have not established clear accountability and metrics for getting the attending physician to complete it in a timely fashion. The author recommends that you establish your meds rec process and ensure physician accountability well in advance of CPOE activation. In addition, one must provide ongoing monitoring and optimization ever after.
  – Another variation that one must understand is the concept of multi-physician meds rec. The author will discuss that further in Chap. 3. However, a facility should be clear on the scope of meds reconciliation for their project.

- CPOE in the Emergency Department

  – The Emergency Department is the front door for most acute care hospitals in the United States, and CPOE creates many opportunities. Many facilities utilize the ED as a pilot unit for CPOE, since it has a defined set of providers and typically starts from a paper MAR (medication administration record). In regards to scope, "Will the ED be the pilot unit for CPOE?" is an important consideration for the executive team. In addition, if you do pilot in the ED, what about admitting doctors who come to the ED?
  – Moreover, the ED physicians should have few verbal orders and no telephone orders. The hospital typically contracts with them, and can incorporate CPOE into their performance metrics. However, the team must provide appropriate order set content for the management of ED patients and an efficient ordering

process. Important metrics for the ED include the time from patient arrival to physician engagement, patient arrival to discharge home, and patient arrival to admission if inpatient care is the result.

- Patient summary views
  - When doing CPOE, physicians like to be able to see a quick snapshot of their patients. The current EMR may already have one or more summary views that bring various elements together onto one view. One should assess whether the current views available will be sufficient for physicians doing CPOE. Typically, the EMR vendor can provide suggestions based on other clients who have already implemented CPOE.
- Ordering processes
  - **Scope of CPOE orders**: The author once consulted on a project in which the client wanted to have the physicians do inpatient CPOE only for laboratory and radiology and not for medications and other orders. This would have created a process in which physicians would be constantly moving between the paper and online chart as they place orders. While this actually might improve throughput in the short term in the ED setting, we would not support fragmenting workflow in this way for inpatients. We believe that one should be giving physicians context during the ordering process and fragmenting the orders does not seem consistent with that effort, or useful to achieving long-term CPOE success. The author passed on this project, as he believes that CPOE should be an all-out effort to create seamless ordering processes with very few exceptions that he will discuss.
  - **Non-formulary meds**: While patients may be taking any of the numerous medications on the market, the hospital pharmacy may have a limited formulary available for its inpatients. Therefore, the team will need to understand how to display only formulary items for inpatient orders, as well as a strategy to allow physicians to convert non-formulary home medications into active hospital orders. Most EMR also provide reference tools online for many medications.
  - **Telephone and verbal orders**: Since telephone and verbal orders are a reality of hospital care, the project must include processes to allow telephone and verbal orders. We will discuss these further in the next Chap. 3.
  - **Co-signature of orders**: The EMR should have some mechanism to ensure that doctors can subsequently sign orders that they give verbally or over the phone. Ideally, this should be an electronic signature with the system "pushing" orders to sign to the physician. Therefore, the CPOE project needs to include a mechanism for electronic signature in its scope. A CPOE metric would be the percentage of telephone/verbal orders with physicians sign within 24 and 48 h, depending on local medical staff bylaws requirements.
  - **TPN (total parenteral nutrition)**: TPN orders are complex and the physician often customizes them for each patient on a daily basis. Modern day CPOE systems should be able to provide solutions for ordering TPN online. Some

medical staffs delegate TPN orders to the pharmacy department, while others keep TPN on preprinted forms.

- **Prescription writing/e-Prescribing**: As physicians discharge patients from the Emergency Department or following an inpatient stay, they will need to provide prescriptions to the patient. Project scope should indicate whether physicians will handwrite patient prescriptions, or the project team will provide an electronic solution. The project team should spell out if prescription printing and/or e-Prescribing will be in scope for the CPOE initiative. The Emergency Department is often an ideal place to start prescription printing and e-Prescribing due to the volume of new prescriptions.
- **Special Orders and Chemotherapy**: The project team should understand how the CPOE system manages orders such as dialysis and chemotherapy. While most EMR vendors will accommodate hemodialysis and chemotherapy protocols, they may require add-on modules or additional design and build time. Therefore, it is advisable that the team make this decision early as to whether physicians will place such orders from pre-printed order sheets or in electronic format. The author would not recommend allowing physicians to handwrite them without some pre-printed template.

- Physician documentation in ED and inpatient

  - Many CPOE projects have not included electronic physician documentation within their scope. The author has found, to the contrary, that physicians adopt online documentation very rapidly when coupled with the CPOE activation. However, there is a strategy that will increase success, and accounted for physicians voluntarily doing over 1.5 million electronic notes at AHS in 2011.
  - The author has found that structured electronic documentation empowers physicians as long as they have the ability to personalize their experiences. He recommends two major elements that will increase your success for physicians voluntarily adopting online notes: grow it virally and combine it with near-time scanning of the paper chart. Since we mentioned AHS above, we will use it as a case study.

Long before Meaningful Use, the team believed that physicians could gain adoption of electronic notes by using a viral marketing approach: find some early adopters to build the business case around personal efficiency then let organic growth occur. Therefore, the they introduced structured electronic notes in October 2008, prior to the initial CPOE pilots in May and June 2009. They utilized our vendor's templates, and added some custom-coded smart templates to add auto-population of data elements that the physicians were already using in their daily Progress Notes. This included T_{max} (the highest temperature in the past 24 h), latest vital signs (while maintaining one-click access to all vital signs from within the note), lists of problems and diagnoses, and laboratory results including bedside blood sugars. Over the past few years, the team has added imaging "Impressions," microbiology summaries, pathology reports, and I & Os (intake and output calculations). Physicians can save pre-completed templates and utilize personal macros as well.

In areas like the ED, the team created "required fields" for the visit diagnosis, which ensures that the visit note meets profession and billing requirements. In the ED, they started with templates based on presenting complaints, and have done little modification to these. They did allow the optional use of speech recognition software, though few use it today. However, one may make the case that it provides a more narrative result than templates for items such as History of Present Illness, Impression and Plan. A handful of ED's do utilize scribes, but this does often delay the completion of the notes rather than enhance them (and creates the need for clear policy as discussed in Chap. 3). We find it quite humorous today now that all of the AHS emergency department documentation is electronic. Previously, the ED physicians were very committed to their paper templates, which allowed them rapid documentation and billing efficiencies, while creating a visit record that other physicians could barely interpret. Today, many of our ED physicians report that it is quicker and easier for them to see a patient that returns to the ED, since they, themselves, can better understand the story of the prior visit from the electronic note than the older paper templates.

AHS added near-time scanning of the paper record as part of the scope of CPOE and it proved a critical success factor for the project as well as for moving physicians to electronic documentation. In addition, it helps the physicians to increase their personal efficiency. The author will discuss the mechanics of this below. However, the goal is to have the entire chart digitalized so that the physician has a complete picture of the patient, whether at the bedside, or viewing the EHR remotely. The efficiency comes as physicians no longer spend time looking for charts, competing with others for the chart, and can review scanned paper notes more quickly than even flipping through pages. Moreover, when the physician no longer goes to a paper chart for any information, it becomes easier to complete an online Progress Note than to look for a paper form to complete. This effectively makes the electronic note the "path-of-least-resistance."

Today, AHS brings new hospitals live from completely paper-based physician workflow to CPOE and electronic documentation with much less physician resistance. They do not prohibit handwritten notes, but the physicians quickly see the benefits of electronic documentation not only for efficiency, but also for more effective physician-to-physician communication and handoffs.

In addition, we teach both ED and inpatient physicians to place orders from within their documentation. This creates valuable timestamps within the notes, and allows all users to get a clear picture of the physician's medical decision-making process.

There can be a downside, however, to electronic templates, as they reveal the heart of some providers. Once live, the HIM (Health Information Management) team and the medical staff should police the process of physicians copying each other notes, using excessive documentation of needless words, or creating inaccurate documentation through mindless use of macros and canned phrases. A real example from several years ago was the description of a patient pharmacologically paralyzed, on a ventilator, and in a drug-induced coma. The physician's canned phrase read, "The patient is alert and oriented." Always remember, the problem is the heart of the documenter and not solely problem with the technology.

- Speech recognition software

  – If the project team determines to include online documentation in scope, then they should consider the option of speech recognition software as well. In the case of physician documentation, the "history of present illness" within the History and Physical Examination report as well as the "hospital course" within the Discharge Summary both lend themselves to narrative structure. While the providers should use structured elements for the Diagnosis and Problem lists as well as orders, there are also opportunities for providers to add narrative commentaries to the Assessment and Plan of documents. The combination of structure and speech recognition can allow providers to add more contexts to their documentation.

- Transcription

  – Since most hospitals already offer transcription with dictation for documents such as History and Physical, Consultation Reports, Operative Reports and Discharge Summary, the consideration for CPOE is around whether physicians will move these reports to structured documentation, and whether providers may dictate daily progress notes. In addition, hospitals now have the option to add "back-end" speech recognition (i.e. provider dictates, voice recognition software transcribes draft document, and transcriptionist performs final edit) to their transcription system. This will only cut costs if that organization negotiates better transcription fees with their transcription vendor, or can perform more transcription per employee if in house.

- Scanning of paper records into EMR

  – As mentioned above under physician documentation, hospitals should strongly consider adding near-time scanning to the scope of their CPOE project. If the paper chart no longer contains orders, physician documentation or nursing/ancillary documentation, then scanning the remaining paper will allow the providers to manage their orders remotely with no gaps in critical results or documentation. The author recommends that one support this by also removing all chart binders and using a clipboard with a front cover, once you start scanning. This serves as another visual anchor to remind the users to go to the EMR and not the paper chart. He also recommends that one use the clipboard only as a location for patient labels, consents that have not yet been fully completed, and forms that remain on paper (e.g. Living Wills, chemotherapy orders, ambulance sheets) until the facility scans them. Moreover, the hospital unit clerk (HUC) should no longer place blank order forms and Progress Note forms on the clipboard. The hospital should avoid printing anything (e.g. lab or imaging reports) that is already in the EHR. This is the time to get all end-users going to the EMR and not the clipboard.

  – At AHS, the team brought near-time scanning live 2 weeks prior to the CPOE go live. Because orders and progress notes were still on paper, the HIM (Health Information Management) department typically had 26 pages of paper to scan daily for each patient. Depending on the unit, they would scan two to four times a day. While the HIM department owns scanning, most sites put scanners on each nursing unit and direct the HUC to scan, with HIM staff overseeing the quality of scanning through audits. Once CPOE went live, the typical scanning volume fell to zero to two (0–2) pages per patient per day as order sheets and Progress Notes went electronic except for orders still on paper (e.g. hemodialysis, chemotherapy) and the occasional handwritten Progress Note.

– Handwriting a Progress Note requires the physician to get the form, write the note, and then place it on the clipboard. The physician still needs to access the electronic record to review orders, results and others' notes. Therefore, many physicians quickly move to online documentation.

– The other benefits of starting scanning 2 weeks before CPOE activation are less obvious, but valuable. First, it makes a clear statement to all end-users that CPOE is moving forward. Second, it gets all the users on the EMR and assures that they can log on and navigate through the EHR. Thirdly, it determines if you have deployed enough devices on the clinical units to accommodate all the users during the peak rounding times. The facility should be able to see an ROI (return on investment) of moving users to the electronic chart and minimizing pages of the patient's record that HIM (Health Information Management department) must collect, scan, index and perform quality assurance. The facility must include the cost of scanners and should acquire some temporary workers to help with scanning during the transition from initial scanning through the first few days of CPOE activation. A metric for scanning is the number of pages of paper per patient per day.

• Clinical decision support

– The author will discuss clinical decision support (CDS) in later chapters. However, he recommends that the team determine the number of CDS alerts that they will include in the initial scope. He recommends that they understand major patient safety opportunities and select six to ten CDS alerts that will get providers engaged in understanding alerts, without over-taxing them early in the process. Some common alerts that physicians understand are around the avoidance of digoxin in the face of electrolyte imbalances, potentially lethal drug combinations, use of anticoagulants in the face of excessive anticoagulation, and warning on certain renally excreted drugs in the face of acute or chronic renal failure. Metrics include number of CDS medication alerts per 100 medication orders and the percentage of alerts in which providers cancel, modify or supplement an order rather than override the alert.

• Code Blue and Rapid Response Teams

– Code Blue is a common term US hospitals use for sudden cardiopulmonary arrest while rapid response teams typically respond to patients who are deteriorating and are at risk for arrest. The author recommends that the project team examine workflows for each, including early warning techniques (such as rules and alerts), and include these in the scope of CPOE. On typically see Code Blue orders as documentation and allow these to remain on paper or as electronic forms. An organization may want to measure the incidence of Code Blues or inhospital mortality as CPOE metrics.

- Anesthesia Information Management System

  - Anesthesiologists have managed their intra-operative documentation for over a century on paper. Their intra-operative records include:

    ○ Common operating room events:

      Anesthesia start time,
      Anesthesia induction time,
      Incision time,
      Surgery stop time,
      Time out of the operating room, and
      Arrival to the post anesthesia care unit/PACU;

    ○ Physiological monitoring (e.g. vital signs, oxygen saturation),
    ○ Intravascular fluid and blood administration,
    ○ Induction medications, and
    ○ Anesthesia administrations:

      Oxygen and nitrous oxide flows, and
      Delivery of IV/inhaled anesthesia/analgesia agents

  - The paper record is often a silo for important information and data such as normally found on the eMAR (electronic medication administration record) and the ongoing calculation of the I & O's (intake and output volumes).
  - Most U.S. hospitals do not have an electronic Anesthesia Information Management System, and therefore remain on the paper Anesthesia Record. When they do, medication and I & O's should flow seamlessly into the appropriate portions of the EMR.
  - If the Anesthesia Record remains on paper for the CPOE project, the author recommends that you still keep pre-operative and PACU processes in scope for CPOE. That means that anesthesiologists will need to utilize CPOE for their pre-operative orders as well as for all the orders in the PACU following surgery. He also recommends that if the anesthesiologist is administering the pre-operative antibiotics, that he documents it on the inpatient eMAR. This will allow better timing for the nurse administering any post-operative antibiotics 8–12 h later.

- Problem List maintenance

  - The Problem List is an excellent communication tool within the EHR, enhancing physician documentation, communication and for helping to optimize clinical decision alerts. The author recommends that physician own the Problem List and its maintenance, and not nursing. Physicians should be able to view and update problems during the ordering and documentation processes. While CDS may suggest to the physician, the inclusion of new problems (such as adding diabetes if the patient is on insulin or has persistent hyperglycemia), the author does not recommend that one automatically add problems as a byproduct of the use of order sets, or other schemes that do not require a physician's confirmation. Otherwise, one will be building long problem lists with no motivation for physicians to review and maintain them. The author does recommend that you utilize CDS to remind physicians when they have not addressed that Problem List during the hospital stay. A metric for Problem List would be percentage of charts in which physicians have documented active problems, or the absence of problems.

- Incentives and CME
  - A final consideration for scope is to include incentives for physicians to adopt CPOE. This could include CME for review of evidence-based content, for attending CME presentations and for training that leads to adoption of evidence-based order sets. The hospital must provide any incentives to all members of the medical staff equally. Planning must occur to offer CME or to budget for other incentives.

As the hospital leadership determines scope of the project, the project manager will work to determine an appropriate timeline and resources. Whether you implement CPOE at one hospital or many hospitals, you will need to have a defined project plan to implement successfully. Fortunately, at AHS, the team had a dedicated project manager, and used a repeatable process to implement multiple times. Chapter 4 will address this topic with more detail.

2.6 Key Points

- Provide a clear vision statement/concept for the project
- Articulate the vision at every event/opportunity
- Use a visual anchor to communicate the vision
- Use the vision for all course corrections
- Wear the vision on your sleeve
- Build an effective plan to fulfill the vision
- Have a content team separate from the IT team
- Define a change control process for managing content
- Allow physician review of order set content at every juncture
- Consider scope that automates physicians' workflow rather than only the ordering process.
- Consider opportunities to move behavior in multiple areas, not just orders.
- Use pre and post-CPOE metrics to demonstrate value and define success.

2.7   Fingernails on the Chalkboard

- **Lack of a central, unifying vision**
  You need to have a vision you can articulate at every level of the organization and with enough authority to overcome the noise of competing priorities. An executive, preferably the CEO or Board, must own and communicate it.
- **Vision statement that only provides value to the organization and not the end-users**
  The vision must provide a strong business case at every level. End-users, including physicians, will act on what provides them value, and are not as strong in their support of projects that value the organization without providing some personal value. Patient safety alone cannot drive the adoption. The end-users also need to see new efficiencies (or similar reward) for their efforts.
- **"The Joint Commission (or CMS, Corporate, etc.) is making us do this!"**
  Organizations that do not provide a clear vision with defined value statements will move into the victim role as its end-user repeat any of these mindless mantra that fail as effective motivators.
- **Absence of a visual anchor**
  A visual anchor, tied to the vision, provides a simple reminder to all of the importance of seeing the project completed. CPOE is a complex project, so a visual anchor helps to keep everyone focused on the reason we are going through this massive change.
- **Absence of a statement of work (scope)**
  Without a clear statement of work on the front end, the organization will not complete the project on time, on budget, or with significant benefit. By clearly defining scope at the start, the team can better project the timeline and resources for success and avoid costly scope creep later.
- **Senior executives not leading the project**
  Organizations always have competing projects. All projects have risks and challenges. The project with the highest level of senior support will always receive priority when competing interests arise, as they always do. CPOE is a major change initiative for an organization, affecting almost every person in a hospital. Having the CEO lead at every occasion sends a clear message of the importance of the project and the commitment for project success.
- **Senior executives multi-tasking or absent during project meetings and major events**
  As in any other leadership, the team watches what the senior leadership does. If the senior leaders lack full engagement, the rest of the team loses its confidence of their support. The executive, who is distracted, such as reading e-mail during a CPOE meeting, sends a conflicting message that this project does not have high priority at the facility.
- **Having the IT team own content**
  CPOE teams chronically underestimate the amount of effort to complete the content. Leaders tend to draft CPOE implementation timelines in stone and not recognize the

importance that content be complete and up to date. It is always best to have a dedicated content team that works independently of the implementation team and are not distracted by last minute IT issues as the activation date approaches.

- **Not having identified physician resources with the time to participate**
  Most CPOE teams have an identified physician, but few have a physician with the time to commit to project success. I have seen many failing CPOE projects that have a roster of physicians on the project who are essentially unengaged. The other risk is the partially engaged physician, who is making recommendations with only peripheral knowledge of the project.

Chapter 3
Leadership and Governance

Abstract The author discusses the importance of developing a leadership structure for your CPOE project. He also lays out the many policies and procedures that a hospital should contemplate as they prepare for their CPOE deployment. The hospital should determine early in their project as to whether to require physicians to comply with mandatory training and CPOE use.

> *Effective leadership is not about making speeches or being liked; leadership is defined by results not attributes.*
>
> *– Peter Drucker*[1]

Leadership expert John C. Maxwell[2] teaches, "Everything rises and falls on leadership." The leadership and governance of a project like CPOE determines how you execute against the vision as well as how you manage obstacles along the way. While many different governance models are possible, you will need to select one that will work with your organizational culture to achieve results. Whenever possible, do not recreate the wheel, but rather use existing structures that you know have worked in the past for success. However, in many cases, this is an opportunity for you to introduce a new model in order to minimize obvious risks.

In the early 2000s, the author assessed an academic hospital that not only wanted to do CPOE, but also had plans to build a new hospital in the subsequent 5 years. The executive team had a decision-making model that each of the C-Suite leaders individually confessed was not working for them. In seeking further clarity, the team discovered that they would tackle big decisions with a consensus-driven mindset, and often process a major decision for 4–5 months, at which time the CEO would commonly step in and make a unilateral decision. It was apparent that one could not drive a 10-month CPOE project with their model of decision-making. They needed a leadership and governance model in which they could process options, make decisions and move on rapidly.

---

[1] Drucker P. BrainyQuote.com, Xplore Inc. 2011. http://www.brainyquote.com/quotes/quotes/p/peterdruck121706.html. Accessed 10 Aug 2011.

[2] John C. Maxwell, author of numerous books on Leadership. www.johnmaxwell.com.

P.A. Smith, *Making Computerized Provider Order Entry Work*,
Health Information Technology Standards,
DOI 10.1007/978-1-4471-4243-0_3, © Springer-Verlag London 2013

As a result, the project team designed a governance model that would lever-age existing committees, build momentum and have the leadership make difficult decisions on a biweekly basis. Three existing committees, IT (technology team), clinical advisory (nursing and ancillaries) and physician advisory (medical staff), would meet separately on a biweekly basis and to ensure they were hitting the milestones on the project plan. On the opposite week, the CPOE Cabinet would meet, review the project and resolve any outstanding decisions or issues arising from the three committees. The executive sponsor chaired the Cabinet, whose membership included the C-Suite executives and two members of each commit-tee. The Cabinet had one guiding principle: the Cabinet would resolve any issues or conflicts arising from any of the three committees in the preceding 2 weeks. If the Cabinet could not come to a decision during the course of the meeting, then the executive sponsor (and Chair) would make a final, binding decision at the conclusion of the meeting.

The Cabinet structure kept the team and the project moving forward. At the first meeting, the executive sponsor had one decision to make. Subsequently, the committees or the Cabinet made the remaining decision. The leadership team was able to move the project forward and move from an unsuccessful consensus model to one of decisive leadership, not only for CPOE, but also for their later building project.

For a multi-hospital health system, the AHS team had to build a governance model that would allow input from each hospital, while keeping the project on track. The health system already had an existing Corporate Clinical Council and the Corporate IT Council as decision-making boards in their respective areas (Fig. 3.1).

The need therefore was to develop leadership groups that could quickly move executive-level decision-making on a monthly basis between the quarterly councils' meetings.

The Corporate Chief Information Officer (Corporate CIO), Corporate Chief Medical Officer (CMO), Chief Medical Information Officer (CMIO), Chief Clinical Information Officer (CCIO) and Chief Information Officer (CIO) made up the CPOE Steering Committee. Non-voting members included the Project Manager, Medical Director and Clinical Applications Director. This was a new committee for the organization. The Steering Committee owned project timeline, scope and resourcing, and met monthly. The CMIO authored the initial charter that clarified the vision, methodologies and assumptions for the project and served as executive sponsor. The Steering Committee served as the mastermind group for the project. It was important that all members contributed to the product.

The Corporate IT Council serves as a governance board over IT operations and approves the overall budget. This was not a new group for the project. It includes the IT executive team as well as regional and divisional CEOs. The CMIO provides monthly updates to this group.

Through the years, the author has found that the actual components of the gover-nance structure are not as important as the various functions that need to occur. In a single hospital organization, the structure is simpler, though the decisions are just as

Fig. 3.1 Example of a CPOE governance model

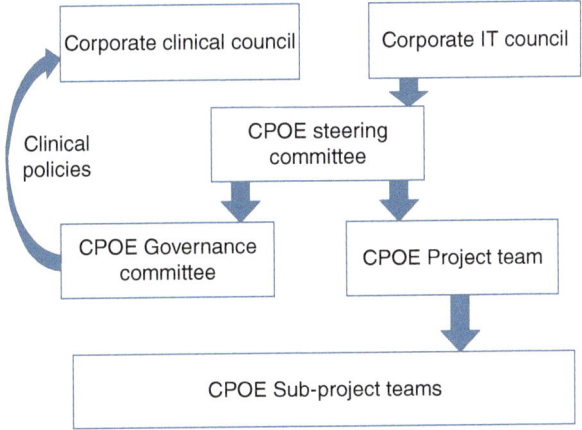

complex. There needs to be a commitment to timeline, resources and a commitment to a defined scope. With a single hospital or small multi-hospital system, the author recommends that you include more local physician participation in the process. In the larger health system, you may need to be creative in your physician engagement plan. If you require physician participation from each hospital, the group becomes too large and unwieldy.

Regardless of size and complexity, the organization should commit to a minimum of specific policies that help avoid confusion in key areas. It is advantageous that you address and formalize your policies before the physicians place their first CPOE orders. Once live on CPOE, you will likely find new opportunities to address other processes with specific policies and procedures.

3.1   CPOE Policies

Through the years and many prior projects, the author has experienced issues with hospitals and medical staffs agreeing to best practices on the front end, then deciding not to follow them once the system is live. Moreover, if dealing with more than one facility, one can anticipate there will be processes that you will need to standardize in order to be successful across multiple facilities. While single facilities may be able to leverage existing structure to create new policies and procedures, a larger system should establish a CPOE Governance Committee to fulfill this role. Typically, one should include the voting members of the CPOE Steering Committee in addition to one C-Suite Executive (CEO, CFO, CMO, CNO or COO) represented each of your hospitals. The purpose of this group is to originate draft policies that all the hospitals would agree to follow – those that are non-negotiable. The group would then forward their approved draft policies to the corporate committee or structure, which owns clinical processes, for review and approval before moving them on to the CEO/Board for final signature.

Typically, the members of the CPOE governance group take their role seriously. They actively discuss, debate and approve multiple policies and procedure that may address the following questions:

- Is CPOE mandatory?
- Is training mandatory?
- When is CPOE required, and what are the exceptions?
- When are verbal or telephone orders appropriate?
- What is the process for entering verbal or telephone orders?
- What is the role of rounding nurses or scribes?
- What is the process for the reconciliation of the patient's medications (i.e. Meds Rec)?

Moreover, the reader will find that the answers to these questions allow the leadership to determine and reinforce the guiding principles of a CPOE initiative.

3.1.1   Is CPOE Mandatory?

The author recommends beginning with an overall policy that doctors taking care of inpatients at our hospitals must use CPOE and the scenarios during which physicians could give orders verbally or over the phone to a nurse. This is where the health system's vision determines the process. With patient safety the reason for CPOE, it would not be reasonable to allow physicians to opt-out of it and continue to hand write their orders. In addition, the author's research of prior CPOE sites compared sites that had gone all at once ("big bang") versus unit by unit or a few physicians at a time. He saw that the hospitals that had deployed in a "big bang" model had rapid adoption and minimal physician resistance, while the latter model created a precarious model of dual processes with some orders on CPOE and some orders on paper. With the latter case, leadership often reports the many risks of important orders falling through the cracks. Moreover, once the leadership accepts voluntary CPOE as the norm, they experience more resistance from the medical staff when they ask them to set the bar higher.

However, if you are putting in a completely new system, you might consider starting with a pilot in a single nursing unit, such as in the Emergency Department (ED) as a "small test of change," in addition to the validation of your system design and build. The benefit of the ED is that it is mainly a self-contained unit with well-defined users. There you can implement CPOE orders, perfect stat turn-around times for lab and radiology, and implement an electronic medication administration record (eMAR). Moreover, you will have a great laboratory for implementing your change management plan, overcoming resistance and negativity, and fine-tuning your content and key workflows. The author's experience has also been that the high volume of the ED leads the doctors and nurses to rapid adoption and competency. Every encounter includes orders, a medication history and interventions. The users will be highly motivated to help iron out the medication administration process and other key workflows.

One caution, however, is that there are nursing units in hospital that one should avoid as potential CPOE pilots. The medical/surgical (med/surg) unit has too much fluctuation in patient flow and physician participation. Even though a hospital may dedicate such a unit to a service line such as orthopaedics, there will still be multiple doctors contributing to orders through consultations. One should avoid a situation in which nurses are managing similar orders across two platforms – paper and electronic. The main consequences are nurses dealing with duplicate orders across the two, as well as missing orders in the confusion.

The other unit to avoid as a pilot is behavioral health or psychiatry. While this represents a unit with minimal fluctuation in users, it typically is not a credible example for the rest of the hospital. This unit has unique individuals and workflows. The author's experience is that it often is slow at adoption and sets a poor example for initial CPOE success.

3.1.2 Is Training Mandatory?

In his career, the author has seen both mandatory training in addition to various combinations of prescribed/suggested schemes. His observation is that physician acceptance and efficiency is often directly proportional to the physician's training effort. In other words, if you like to see physicians struggle with CPOE after go live, then do not have them train to a level of competency. However, the author will discuss more on training in a later chapter.

3.1.3 When Is CPOE Required, and What Are the Exceptions?

Early in the project, an entity needs to have frank discussion about when CPOE is required, and when it is optional. The author typically works through this exercise to determine this by venue, by process and by context:

- Which units will be doing CPOE, both during pilots and once deployed?
- Will the Emergency Department (ED) physicians do CPOE?
- Will the ED nurses chart mediation administration on an electronic medication administrative record (eMAR) or on paper?
- Will physicians order outpatient tests/labs using CPOE?
- Will surgeons place Pre-Admission Testing (PAT) orders using CPOE?
- Will surgeons place Pre-Operative orders (i.e. the orders necessary to prepare a patient for an operation on the morning of surgery) using CPOE or on paper, and if the latter, whose responsibility is it to enter those orders into the EMR?
- What is your process for accepting "direct admission" orders, for patients coming directly from another location such as physician office, urgent care clinic or other health care facility when the admitting doctor is initiating that transfer/admission and bypassing the ED?
- Will the behavioral health or psychiatric physicians enter orders using CPOE?
- Who will enter/record intra-operative orders?

- What is your downtime process for entering orders?
- What is your uptime process for orders following a downtime?
- At go-live, what is your process for back-loading existing orders on current inpatients?
- When is it appropriate for a physician to give a verbal or a telephone order?
- Who can accept a verbal or telephone order and what is the process for entering it electronically?
- What is your process for handling CDS (clinical decision support) alerts that occur during a non-CPOE order process?
- Are there any types of orders that are exceptions to CPOE?
- Are there any specific scenarios that you plan to exclude from CPOE?
- What are your long-term plans for remedying your short-term decisions?
- How will you enter and reconcile the patient's home medications?
- How will you order and communicate the patient's discharge medications?
- How will you handle discharge prescriptions from the ED and from the inpatient unit?

3.1.4 When Are Verbal or Telephone Orders Appropriate?

In the United States, many physician care for patients in hospital as well as having private office practices. Therefore, it is crucial that the organization determine early in the process the policy and procedure for allowing verbal and telephone orders. Though no one has established a "tolerance level" for verbal or telephone levels, industry organizations in the U.S. have set clear goals for their purposes of certification and recognition. The opinion commonly cited in the field is that providers should directly place 94 % of the orders into the CPOE system, thus defining a tolerance of 6 % for verbal/telephone orders. HIMSS Analytics, of the Health Information Management Systems Society, sets a minimal goal of 90 % for organizations they recognize for their top tier for the United States EMR Adoption Model. The Leapfrog Group, the leading business organization committed to CPOE adoption states as its standard: "Assure that physicians enter at least 75 % of medication orders via a computer system that includes prescribing-error prevention software; and demonstrate, via a test, that their inpatient CPOE system can alert physicians to at least 50 % of common, serious prescribing errors."[3] The author's personal recommendation is an initial implementation goal of 100 % of providers performing CPOE with a verbal/telephone incidence rate of less than 20 %, then work through processes and adoption to reduce that within 1–2 years to less than 6–10 %.

The author recommends that each organization clearly determine appropriate conditions for verbal/telephone orders. Three common ideas are:

- A physician may give a verbal order when scrubbed for surgery or otherwise physically unable to enter the order (e.g. scrubbing for surgery)

---

[3] *Factsheet: Computerized Physician Order Entry.* http://www.leapfroggroup.org/media/file/FactSheet_CPOE.pdf

- A physician may give verbal orders during emergency resuscitation efforts (in the U.S. known as "Code Blue", such as during cardiopulmonary resuscitation)

  – This reasonably includes any situation in which the physician's active intervention/attention to the patient precludes her ability to directly perform CPOE and it is reasonable for the nurse to accept a verbal order (Example would be the physician applying pressure to tamponade bleeding or actively assessing a patient during a critical juncture.)

- A physician may give a telephone order when off-campus (i.e. not in hospital) and does not have ready access to device capable of performing CPOE. The common example is a physician attending her child's sporting event.

The key, in these cases, is that the organization sets CPOE as the standard order entry paradigm yet empower the physician to make a judgment when a verbal or telephone order is appropriate. To obtain its goal of achieving significant CPOE success, the organization must provide near real-time data of an individual's CPOE rates. While the majority of providers have no difficulty in achieving 90–95 % CPOE rates, the organization must actively address those providers that are performing below the 80 % level and remove obstacles. The author's one word of caution is that one must not assume that low performance always represents an attitude against CPOE success. However, the leadership should promote the value of CPOE and CDS and help to remove real and perceived obstacles from the outliers.

3.1.5   What Is the Process for Entering Verbal or Telephone Orders?

With improved patient safety as the primary outcome of CPOE, the organization will implement clinical decision support (CDS) rules and alerts into the ordering process. These alerts give immediate feedback for the ordering provider. The author's experience is that CDS should influence around 10 % of the medication orders in the system. This will go down over time as doctors move to more structured order sets and repetitive processes. In the world of hand-written orders, CDS is a manual process that may result in a cascade of phone calls more than an hour after the provider places the order:

Dr. Jones handwrites six medication orders and places the chart next to the clerk where it sits until the clerk pulls the order sheet from the chart and transmits in information to the pharmacist. The pharmacist then proceeds to assess legibility of the orders, completeness (med name, route, dose, frequency and duration) and if possible, proceeds with transcribing the orders into the pharmacy system. Throughout the process, the pharmacist is determining the "will of the physician" to the best of her ability, despite barriers such as poor handwriting and incompleteness of the details. Finally, as the pharmacist enters each order, CDS alerts may appear, and the pharmacist addresses and overrides based on experience, and occasionally on "assuming what Dr. Jones would do in this case." If the process is unsuccessful, due to illegibility, incompleteness or an alert that needs medical decision-making, the pharmacist either puts the process on hold and attempts to contact Dr. Jones directly, or contacts the nurse to contact Dr. Jones. Through this process, however, the first dose of that new medication is on hold, such as delaying an antibiotic or other time-sensitive intervention for the patient's treatment. Eventually, the nurse contacts Dr. Jones who provides clarity to the order. Often this process adds considerable delay to the medication process.

In the CPOE process, the system requires completeness of the order (e.g. required fields for route, dose and frequency) and maintains legibility. As the provider enters the order, the system is analyzing for drug-drug interactions, drug-allergy issues and checking the appropriateness of the dose amount, based on factors such as age and weight. When alerts occur, the provider has immediate feedback from CDS. She makes a clinical determination within the context of the medical decision-making process as to heed the alert (cancel the med, modify the order or perhaps order some additional intervention, such as a laboratory test to monitor for problems with the medication.) or overrides the alert (and document the medical decision-making rationale). In the case of CDS, the order processes in a clean, complete and seamless manner, and is immediately available to the pharmacist to verify (i.e. ensure that the medication is appropriate in the context of other medications as well as the age and weight of the patient – a second pair of eyes on the process).

Remembering that the provider will likely accept CDS recommendations in one of every ten medications orders, the system design should allow the medication process to leverage your investment in patient safety. Therefore, only licensed clinical healthcare workers responsible for the medication process (such as nurses and pharmacists), should enter medication orders into the CPOE system. When the provider is not the one entering the order directly, you no longer have the medical decision-making to order authoring process connected, thus creating opportunities for the process to fail. Therefore, the industry has adopted a process known as "order read-back" to add an additional level of safety.

The process of order read-back began with handwritten orders and The Joint Commission, the leading health care accreditation body in the U.S. promotes it. In the paper process, a provider speaks an order (as either a "verbal order", i.e. in-person; or a "telephone order" i.e. via telephony) while the nurse actively transcribes the order onto the "source of truth", typically an order sheet. Before the process is considered to consummate a legitimate order, the nurse must "read-back" the complete order(s) to the provider, "from the source of truth", and confirm that the nurse's transcription of the order is complete and fully represents the provider's intent (i.e. the medical decision-making). In this process, the nurse cannot use any intermediate transcription, such as writing the order on a scrap of paper or hand, for later entry into the "source of truth" order sheet.

The "source of truth" in the EMR, is the electronic order. Therefore, the nurse (or pharmacist) should only enter verbal or telephone orders directly into the EMR and perform the read-back with the provider before the order is processed. Using this process of direct order entry with immediate read-back, CDS alerts occur in the same manner as with direct CPOE, and the nurse can discuss the alerts and address them with the provider.

Common variations of this process create issues that dilute the effectiveness of the CPOE system. For example, many organizations rationalize that they "don't want to keep the physician on the phone too long" and therefore promote the nurse writing down the order on a paper order sheet then later entering the order into the EMR and calling the physician if CDS alerts occur and need physician response. While such hospitals do scan and retain the immediate order sheet as an audit trail, the process adds additional failure opportunities into the medication process:

1. Communicates to all that "convenience of the physician" is a higher value than a safer medication process
2. Reintroduces transcription errors into the process, rather than the provider directly entering her orders into the EMR as occurs with CPOE
3. Assumes that all nurses will call a physician back to address CDS alerts rather than taking a "best guess" on how Dr. Jones would have addressed that alert
4. Since the entry of the order is not instantaneous, it inherently adds delays to the administration of the first dose of the medication

While each of the above dilutes the potential safety opportunities of CPOE, the first issue directly reveals the true leadership vision of the initiative. If patient safety is the "true north" principle of a CPOE initiative, then the organization will anchor every process to the safest process, rather than the most convenient process. For example, the author has demonstrated that through remote access, proper training and competency, and with the availability of order sets, most physicians can log in and place orders through CPOE and address the CDS alerts much faster than getting a nurse on the phone, then on a computer, entering the order and read-back. Likewise, the remote CPOE process is more efficient and effective than the workaround of writing phone orders down and later calling back the physician for clarity around CDS alerts. Thoughtful analysis by the organization leadership will determine the direction and path that will be most successful in getting the right medication to the right patient in the shortest time. Moreover, the process creates transparency of which principles the organization values the most.

3.1.6 What Is the Role of Rounding Nurses or Scribes?

In the U.S., some community-based physicians utilize office nurses who perform hospital rounds with them. In the Emergency Department, some ED physicians employ scribes to document their encounters to allow the provider to focus on assessing the patient and performing hands-on procedures. While rounding nurses, by definition, are licensed nurses, scribes are typically college students who do not have extensive clinical experience or credentials. Therefore, a health system should recognize in advance of CPOE which actions each role may perform. Moreover, since the doctor, not the hospital is likely to employee these assistants to the physicians, it is important that the hospital recognizes the need to manage security and electronic credentials on these individuals. Finally, each person must have his own log in and security within the EHR, and never log in using the provider's electronic credentials.

The hospital, therefore, should commit to policy and procedures on credentialing/ certifying these roles, a process to follow when the physician terminates her employees in this role and the management of the assistant's security and privileges within the hospital and more importantly, within the Electronic Health Record (EHR). Finally, the hospital must formally acknowledge the scope that each performs, as well as the limitations.

Most organizations will allow a licensed rounding nurse to receive verbal orders and telephone orders and enter these directly into the CPOE system as long as the nurse complies with verbal order read back. Rounding nurses typically initiate/draft physician Progress Notes, Consultation Notes and possibly History and Physical documentation as long as the physician is actually doing the physical exam and medical decision-making. However, rounding nurses should not be entering verbal orders without direct and immediate read back to the supervising physician. A nurse entering an order otherwise would be practicing beyond the scope of his practice (unless the rounding nurse has credentials as a provider himself, such as an advanced nurse practitioner).

The ED scribe, who is not a nurse, should only interact with the EMR in the presence of the ED physician. The scribe captures documentation as the ED physician "thinks aloud" and is not there to make assessments, examine the patient, suggest diagnoses or orders. Some health systems allow scribes to enter orders that the physician must sign prior to the order processing or transmitting. However, allowing a non-clinical person to enter orders may set up the ED physician to relegate increasing responsibility to the scribe with the potential to compromise patient safety. Most systems choose to limit the scope of scribes to only encounter documentation, and not allow this role any participation in the ordering process. Regardless, the health system or hospital should make these determinations prior to CPOE and ensure that the policies align with the vision of the project.

3.1.7 What Is the Process for the Reconciliation of the Patient's Medications (i.e. Meds Rec or Medication Reconciliation)?

One of the most important foundations of the medication process is the medical decision-making processes regarding the patient's current list of medications each time care moves to a different venue (e.g. from critical care unit to regular nursing unit). In the past decade, the health care industry has put increasing attention on the medication reconciliation process. For successful CPOE, a facility or health system must give thoughtful consideration of the entire medication process, and especially set clear expectation on ownership of the various sub-processes. By clearly setting expectations and maintaining accountability along each step, the health system will experience less chaos in the process and each patient will benefit. The organization should approve a clear and concise policy and procedure around the process, accountability and mechanics of meds rec. While each EMR vendor is different in their meds rec tools, the overall goal is to have the provider safely review and reconcile the patient's current list of medication each time a venue of care changes. Prior to writing a local policy, the organization should clearly understand and document the workflow and functionality of their meds rec tools. However, this is a very important policy to have in place early in your project, so the author will spend some time on the topic.

The foundation for successful medication reconciliation is the medication history itself. In fact, this author, often states that medication reconciliation is a workaround for a broken medication history process.

In the U.S., despite all our automation, the patient is still the "source of truth" for a list of current medications. There is no reliable, complete and up to date repository of current medications for the individual patient.[4] Thus, no one can be sure what medications a provider has prescribed or what the patient actually takes.

Often a patient arrives at hospital confused, in pain or even unaware of a complete list of current medications. Others may be elusive in admitting to a doctor or nurse their non-compliance (either conscious or accidental). We must look to the future for a complete, real-time repository of every patient's current list of medications. When we have access to that database, medication reconciliation will be a redundant concept.

Recently the author started a cause and effect diagram to better clarify the entire medication process and the resultant dissatisfaction that physicians and nurses experience in the process. We show this in Fig. 3.2 below.

One notes on Fig. 3.2 that there are many failure opportunities in the upper right of the cause and effect diagram. These represent the steps and barriers of obtaining and documenting the current list of medications.

Once the nurse or pharmacist has documented the medication history in the EMR, the physician then considers each current medication individually in the process. Considerations include:

- Is this medication still appropriate for the patient at this time?
- Should I order this medication during the current venue of care?
- Should I order this medication with the same route, dose and frequency?
- Should I substitute some other medication for this one?

---

[4] e-Prescribing (the electronic routing of prescriptions from provider to pharmacy) has enabled the pharmacies and pharmacy benefits managers (PBM) to establish a robust database linking chain and independent pharmacies, as well as large medication distribution centers and PBM. Currently their database, incorporating *SureScripts* and *RxHub*, captures about 90 % of the prescribed medications in the U.S. However, patients have other sources of medications, including samples, non-participating pharmacies (both domestic and abroad) in addition to well meaning families and friends. In addition, regional health information organizations (RHIO) and health information exchanges (HIE) improve access to medication histories, but are not the complete "source of truth".

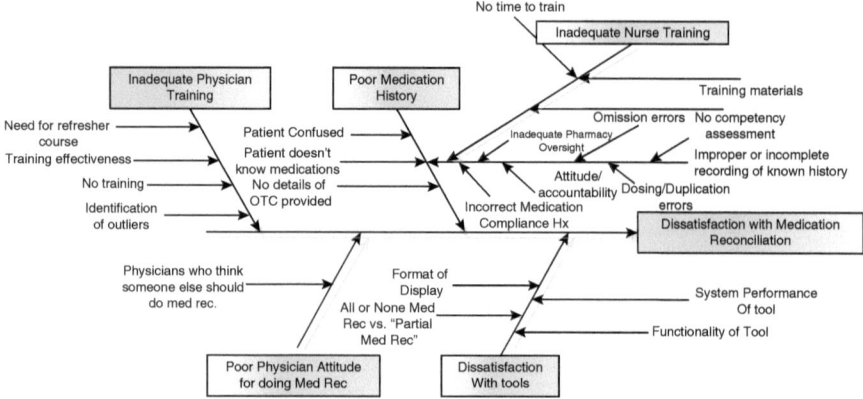

Fig. 3.2 Cause and effect diagram showing reasons for dissatisfaction with medication reconciliation

- Are there any drug-drug, drug-allergy interactions involved?
- Is this medication on the hospital formulary, and if not, what is the best substitute?

Then the physician must decide if she should add one or more additional medications at this time?

When the physician first admits the patient to hospital, this initial consideration of home medications becomes "admission meds rec". Then every time the physician decides a new level of care is appropriate (i.e. transfer from critical care to a regular medical nursing unit), re-review of the home and inpatient medications occurs in the process of "transfer meds rec". Finally, at the conclusion of the hospital stay, the provider determines (through "discharge meds rec") which of the original home meds and the current inpatient medications will comprise the medications the patient will continue at the next venue of care (e.g. at home, at a skilled nursing facility or domiciliary).

Throughout the hospital stay, there may be multiple physicians contributing to the care of the patient. The organization will need to define whether the attending physician has sole responsibility for medication reconciliation or whether multiple physicians may contribute to the process (commonly known as partial or multi-contributor meds rec). Again, the author offers some insight and opinion:

In a hospital environment there are often multiple physicians co-managing the patient. However, it is best to have only one ultimately in charge – the attending physician. Often we hear that the psychiatrist works with the primary care physician to manage the psychotrophic medications and non-psychotrophic medications respectively. In addition, surgeons frequently claim they do not want to take responsibility for medications that some other physician prescribed. From a patient's standpoint, someone has to be in charge and make a timely decision of the medical plan of care.

My recommendation is the attending physician is ultimately in charge of leading the medical team. She should take responsibility to get the input of her consultants in determining the plan.

To our surgeon colleagues, who chose to attend to patients, we tend to explain that medication reconciliation is not about complete familiarity of each medication. However, this should result in the surgeon giving thoughtful review as to whether he should stop any current medications that might interfere with the surgeon's post-operative plan. The surgeon may later choose to consult a medical colleague for complete review of unfamiliar medications. In addition, the latter becomes an opportunity to reduce polypharmacy.[5] Having the attending as the sole owner of medication reconciliation helps to prevent delays as a single physician takes ownership the admission, transfer and discharge process. The patient and her family suffer when the attending communicates the discharge to the patient and then writes an order, "Discharge if OK with Dr. _____" (i.e. one or more consultants on the case), only to have the patient and family waiting hours for the consulting physician(s) to arrive and complete the discharge.

An organization needs to take a definitive stand on the ownership of both the med history process (typically nursing with pharmacist review and oversight) and the meds rec process (typically only providers). The policy should not only include the ownership, but the accountability and the timeliness of completion. A strong, consistent message on this topic will ensure a safer product for patient care.

3.1.8 What Is the Process for Direct Admissions from the Physician's Office to Hospital?

While many countries have office physicians that no longer practice inpatient hospital care, most U.S. hospitals still have many community physicians who decide to admit a sick patient directly to a hospital unit from her office. Prior to CPOE, the physician sends the patient carrying written orders from the office to the hospital. From there the patient goes to the admitting department and sits until a bed is available. Often delays in care results, so this is an opportunity to design a new process.

An organization can leverage workflow redesign, and streamline the direct admission process and back it up with a defined policy and procedure. The author commonly defines the CPOE direct admission process as follows:

- The physician makes a decision to admit
- The physician's office manager contacts the admission coordinator at the hospital, who creates a pre-admission encounter in the EMR. The hospital determines which nursing unit the patient will go and the patient leaves the office for the hospital.
- The physician, who has since seen her next patient, remote accesses into the EMR, finds the new encounter and enters future orders for admission.
- The patient arrives at the hospital and a staff member escorts him to the appropriate nursing unit.
- The admitting nurse confirms the identity of the patient and checks the availability of admission orders (future or planned orders). If both are successful, the nurse escorts the patient to the proper room, and begins the orientation and admission intake process, which includes activating and reviewing the admission orders.

---

[5] Polypharmacy refers to the practice of placing patients on large number of medications, increasing the risk of drug-drug interactions and mishaps.

- As the nurse is obtaining the admission data and information (e.g. reason for admission, allergies, medication history and initial vital signs), the phlebotomist (person who draws blood specimens for the hospital laboratory) arrives and obtains blood specimens.
- When the nurse has completed his assessment, he checks for which medications to administer first, and begins the medication administration process.
- Meanwhile the admission clerk completes the registration process at bedside.
- Once initial medication administration is complete, the patient can proceed for further tests and imaging studies, based on the physician's orders.

Ideally, the team works in parallel and starts initial treatments and interventions within 30 min to an hour. By having a defined workflow and a definitive policy and procedure, the organization can improve such measures as speed to first dose of an antibiotic, and time for nurses to complete the admission process. In addition, prepare to hear the phrase, "That's not how we do it here!"

3.1.9   What Is the Process for Admission from the Emergency Department (ED)?

In the U.S., organizations admit the majority of adult medical patients following initial presentation to the ED. While ED physicians perform immediate assessments and early orders, they typically contact a "Physician on Call" (or the patient's personal physician) from among the medical staff to discuss potential admission to hospital. The emergency departments initially triage and manage their patients through the course of the ED encounter. However, if the ED physician determines a need for inpatient hospitalization and a member of the hospital accepts the admission of the patient, the latter needs to provide admission orders and enter them, as in the case of direct admissions above.

In a significant number of hospitals in the U.S., ED physicians have developed a tradition of writing the initial admission orders on behalf of the admitting physician. The most likely time the ED physician writes these so-called "tuck in" or transition orders is during the nighttime hours. While some consider this advantageous, others consider it inappropriate. The slippery slope of this process is that the hospital typically does not extend admitting privileges to these ED physicians, yet these orders may represent the entire medical care plan until the attending physician sees and examines the patient. During these transition hours, the attending is responsible for the ongoing care of the patient, yet has not really taken the reins of medical decision-making.

Prior to CPOE, the organization should assess the current state of ED admissions and determine whether they are comfortable with the current state or whether they would like to effect change. The author has experienced many hospitals in which the admitting physician writes all admission orders immediately upon notification that the ED physician recommends admission to the hospital. The second variant is when the admitting physician agrees to write the orders, yet does not do it in a timely fashion. This leaves a patient occupying an ED bed with an unclear picture of which physician is actively managing the patient (ED physician or the admitting physician).

If the ED physician is writing the admitting orders, one should make every effort to start dialogue among the ED physicians, the Medical Executive Committee and the hospital executives to create a definitive plan to move toward an end of the practice, except in life-threatening transfers to the critical care unit or the operating room. The ideal time for the medical staff to make this transition is prior to the implementation of CPOE. The other alternative is to transition 3–6 months after the CPOE implementation. The author recommends that the CPOE implementation date is not the day to change the process. While he has seen the rare hospital be successful with this approach, it commonly creates a "blame-game" of CPOE victimhood that becomes a distraction at a time of focus on many other new workflows. The ED physicians, while seeing the current state as customer friendly to the medical staff, also understand that it is more appropriate for the admitting physician to own the medical decision-making and plan of care. The admitting physicians will likely argue that the ED physician has most recently examined the patient and is the best person to make these decisions. The author recommends that you take the position that once the ED and admitting physicians agree that there is a reason to admit, the entire care should immediately transition to the admitting physician. This allows the ED physician to focus on his primary role of running an emergency department. One may want to minimize the number of processes that change on the day of CPOE implementation, and both ED and admitting physicians may polarize on this one. Instead, focus your dialogue on "What is the right thing for patient care?" and make the change independent of your implementation date.

3.1.10 How Do You Manage Standing Orders and Protocols?

When you focus your CPOE project on patient safety, you will also have the opportunity to have discussion and planning around the concepts of standing orders and protocols. Again, this is a topic that your medical staff may have passionate opinions and your nursing staff may have engrained patterns of behavior. Let us start, however, with definitions to distinguish the two:

- Standing orders – orders generically approved by a physician and applied by nursing discretion to an individual patient. Examples include a selection of "as needed orders" such as non-narcotic analgesics, pills that promote sleep, or over-the-counter medications.
- Protocol orders – orders standardized and approved by the governing body that the physician may order, as the indicated protocol, on a specific patient. Nurses thereby follow the orders as the protocol specifies, typically when the patient situation meets defined parameters. Examples include a standard for specific orders to replace potassium or magnesium if blood tests indicate a deficiency of either.

- Policy-driven orders – orders standardized and approved by the governing body that are initiated by the nurse without modification, prior to examination by a physician, to administer care to a patient who presents with a life-threatening or pre-defined situation. Examples of "initiated by policy" orders include:

  - ED triage orders (those immediate interventions which the ED medical director deems necessary to facilitate rapid assessment of patients presenting with life-threatening or common scenarios, such as electrocardiogram for an adult with acute onset of chest pain)
  - Rapid response team orders (orders permitted by a critical care nurse upon emergent assessment of a non-critical care patient with rapid deterioration)
  - Routine newborn orders for unattended deliveries (order for antibiotic eye ointment or vitamin K in the delivery suite).

3.1.11 Standing Orders

For decades, hospitals allowed physicians to create and maintain a list of standing orders. The physician would annually sign a standing order sheet and when a nurse needed something when the physician was not available, she would go to the file cabinet, pull out Dr. Smith's standing orders, and see what was available for giving the patient without contacting the physician directly. However, this situation actually put the nurse in a position of "physician proxy". Since nurses may not order medications on patients specifically, this forced the nurse to function beyond her scope of practice.

In 2008, the Centers for Medicare and Medicaid (CMS, the largest government payor in the U.S.), published in their federal regulations that nurses cannot act on standing orders. According to this CMS communication, however, hospitals could screen patients and administer immunizations for influenza and pneumonia without a physician order. CMS acknowledged this as a safety measure for both the patient and the hospital environment, as long as the patient did not refuse the immunization (and of course, the patient was unimmunized). While standing orders should be a relic of the past, the CPOE team may discover these during the initial assessment and move the hospital to address through specific policy.

3.1.12 Protocol Orders

While standing orders represent those orders available for a nurse to activate with personal discretion on a specific patient, protocol orders allow hospitals to provide standardized solutions to common patient care issues. However, unlike standing orders, a physician (or midlevel provider) must first place the patient on the actual protocol through an order, rather than leaving the ordering to the nurse's discretion. Once the physician has placed the order(s) for a specific protocol for the individual patient, the nurse responds as the patient qualifies for the conditions of the protocol.

For example, Dr. Smith is expecting that his treatment plan may lead to low levels of potassium in the blood, which in itself can cause serious heart dysrhythmias. Therefore, Dr. Smith orders the Potassium Oral Replacement Protocol for the patient. The following morning, a new laboratory (e.g. blood) test demonstrates that the patient's serum potassium is now low. The nurse checks for the physician's order for the potassium replacement protocol. She then accesses the actual protocol orders and selects the right replacement orders based on the clinical finding(s). The EMR specifically identifies a physician order for the protocol. The physician need not sign the subsequent order, since the order was a conditional order, which he specified when placing the order for the defined protocol. However, the hospital's P & T (Pharmacy and Therapeutics) Committee and the Medical Executive Committee (MEC) must approve the standard protocol.

3.1.13   Policy-Driven Orders

Hospitals and medical staffs create policy-driven orders for common situations within hospital. Nurses, under specific policy, initiate these orders, without modification, when a patient specifically meets the conditions of the policy. However, unlike protocol orders, the Joint Commission directs that the physician must subsequently examine the patient, document that exam and sign these orders within 24 h, regardless of any hospital policy that might allow the physician a longer time (e.g. 48 h) to cosign other orders. In contrast to standing orders, the nurse, who initiates policy-driven orders, must elicit all the orders within the available orders under the policy and not "pick and choose" from a menu of orders. The only exception occurs if the policy specifically addresses a life-threatening scenario, such as the application of advanced resuscitation orders for life-threatening cardiac dysrhythmias or circulatory collapse.

As mentioned above, the pediatric department may devise routine newborn orders that the nurse activates upon birth, without variation, on all unattended deliveries. For anything other than these specific orders, the nurse contacts the physician for further direction. Likewise, the ED physicians may approve specific orders initiated upon common presentations to the emergency department, such as electrocardiogram for an adult with chest pain. Again, the nurse must activate all the orders the policy specifies for that presentation without modification or omission. Once the ED physician sees the patient, the nurse may no longer activate additional policy orders, but rather rely on the physician for further orders.

The policy for these orders should specify how the hospital monitors and maintains the medical staff's compliance with the 24-h exam and signoff.

3.2 Physician Leadership

Having physician leadership at the table throughout a CPOE project will add credibility to your initiative. This person brings the mind of the medical end-user to the
table, ensuring:

- That your design has relevance to the physician
- That your training plan is sound
- That your support model is appropriate, and
- That your vision is clear

The physician leader should have a strategic rapport with key medical staff and
hospital leaders, deliver key messages to the medical staff, provide a vision to your
outcomes research and quality, author peer-reviewed journal articles, present region-
ally and nationally and shepherd/engage the hospital Chief Medical Officer (CMO)
on CPOE and EHR topics. We discuss the characteristics and role of physician leaders more in Chap. 5.

3.3 Key Points

- Leadership is key to project success
- The Chief Executive Officer is the best choice to lead CPOE at the hospital level
- A CPOE project should have a defined governance structure
- The CPOE project must align with its vision
- CPOE governance should include specific policies and procedures, which the
  organization deems as "non-negotiable"

3.4 Fingernails on the Chalkboard

- **There is no governance structure for steering and policy-making**
  Effective governance will ensure that the project stays on track and under budget.
  By having well thought out policies, the end-users will be able to concentrate on
  adoption of the CPOE system rather than focusing on ways to maintain the status
  quo. When your health system defines clear direction in these key areas of patient
  care, your physicians and other end-users avoid chaos, confusion and conflict
  that results when you fail to provide specific guidance in these areas. These policies help the end-users to better define their "best practice" workflows and remain
  confident that the organization's leadership, and not the IT department, is clearly
  governing the project.

- **The organization discusses policies, but does not formally approve and publish them**
  Many organizations are well intended and discuss the need for policies, yet fail to formalize them. As a result, departments and users throughout the hospital (and in the case of a health system, across the hospitals) develop unique workflows and achieve various levels of adoption. Not only is it hard to fix this after the fact, but the organization will find it difficult to analyze future changes to the system. When the need arises to modify the design of the CPOE system, the team spends much effort trying to understand the endless workflow variations and the impact these changes might have on the respective end-users. In addition, organizations that define clear policies and enforce them instill a level of confidence to the end-users that these decisions are important.
- **Any governance solely resides in the IT department**
  Having governance reside solely in IT communicates to the end-users that CPOE is a technology that you are forcing on them, rather than a component of the organization's patient safety initiatives.
- **There are no regular governance meetings**
  Leadership makes time for the meetings they feel are most important and communicate otherwise when they repeatedly move or cancel specific meetings.
- **Poor attendance or disengagement at governance meetings**
  See comment above.
- **No policies exist**
  Everything in a hospital begins and ends with a physician order. So changing the way doctors order will change every process in the hospital. Moreover, without consistent policies and procedures in place, the organization will experience variations in adoption, in patient care and in outcomes.
- **Policies do not support the project vision**
  Since the vision of the project determines "true north", the organization will proceed off course if the policies do not align with the stated vision.
- **The organization publishes, but does not operationalize or enforce the policies**
  Organizations that write policies, yet do not enforce them, rarely achieve greatness. Moreover, in times of conflict, they have already demonstrated that they do not follow their policies and therefore have no grounds on which to enforce them. These organizations frequently fail at implementing projects as complex as CPOE. Therefore, it is best to address the problem before a CPOE even begins.
- **The recommended workflow is in contrast to the policies and procedures**
  Whenever this happens, rather early or late in the project, it indicates that the leadership has not clearly distributed and/or communicated the policies. If this happens, one should take a critical look at the project structure and the communication plan.

Chapter 4
Project Management Key Opportunities

Abstract This chapter covers the key considerations a hospital should address in their CPOE project planning. The chapter also discusses key considerations of software capability and functions that affect the hospital's CPOE design. In addition, the author recommends critical success factors for a CPOE pilot.

> *If you fail to plan, you are planning to fail*
> *– Benjamin Franklin, United States Founding Father*

Once senior leadership has committed to the vision of the CPOE project, they assign a project manager who will be dedicated to this project throughout its life cycle. Good project management keeps a CPOE initiative on track, on time and on budget. While the methodology may vary, the organization must first determine a defined scope, develop a timeline then commit the resources for success. This chapter will not replace the need for a competent project manager. Project managers bring discipline and methodology to the project and provide tremendous value. Organizations that scrimp in this area are sure to pay a higher cost of implementing CPOE, in both time and resources.

The author likes to develop CPOE in two steps: the product phase and the implementation phase. The product phase develops the CPOE platform while the implementation phase includes any piloting and rollout of CPOE to the end-users. The two overlap, in an iterative cycle, as the project moves from initial testing, piloting, post-go-live stabilization and ongoing optimization. The author likes to separate change management from project management as well. While project management defines scope, timeline and resourcing, change management drives the people side of the project. He will address change management in Chaps. 5 and 6. This chapter addresses the key points the steering committee and the project manager should address as they begin their CPOE journey.

This is not a comprehensive chapter on CPOE project management. Instead, the author will focus on key questions that the project manager will need to address. In addition, he will list some critical success factors for CPOE. Chapter 1 addressed the scope and high-level timeline of the project. He will also assume that you are working with a commercial EMR vendor, rather than developing your own software.

P.A. Smith, *Making Computerized Provider Order Entry Work*,
Health Information Technology Standards,
DOI 10.1007/978-1-4471-4243-0_4, © Springer-Verlag London 2013

Therefore, he will not discuss detail on how to actually build an EMR for CPOE, but rather highlight several design, build and test steps that the author has seen sites overlook in their CPOE journey.

4.1   The Product Phase

The initial investigation for the project manager is the current state of the EMR platform. Are all the elements built or are components lacking for CPOE success? Key considerations may include:

- What components currently exist in the EMR platform?
- Is the EMR fully integrated or several best of breed applications?
- Does the EMR have a physician-friendly order catalogue?
- Does the EMR have medication integration in place?
- What are the EMR tools for clinical decision support?
- Does the EMR provide electronic documentation tools for providers?
- How do charges drop through orders and documentation?
- Is there a content process for order sets and documentation?
- How do providers maintain problem lists?
- How will providers co-sign verbal and telephone CPOE orders?

The author will discuss each of these topics briefly as they pertain to CPOE. The reader may want to refer to any of the good implementation guides on the market. The organization needs to determine whether they will resource their project with their own employees, have the EMR vendor do most of the work effort, hire third-party consultants, or any combination of these.

4.1.1   What Components Currently Exist in the EMR Platform?

In planning for CPOE, the project team must have a good idea as to what components already exist within the EMR. The author recommends that you look at CPOE beyond just electronic order entry and look for opportunities to automate the physician workflow as you implement CPOE. As you review the inventory of what you have in place, the team begins to document the gap between the current state and the future state. This represents what they will need to design and build in order to automate the workflows that are in scope. Obviously, the organization will need to purchase any modules or additional software necessary to close this gap.

Taking the time to develop a gap analysis between current and future states is important for both system (technology) design as well as workflow (process) design. The author has visited sites pre-implementation and found gaps between what the organization was hoping to accomplish with CPOE and what they had actually purchased from their EMR vendor. Both the healthcare organization and the EMR vendor have a stake in avoiding this unfortunate situation.

4.1.2   Is the EMR Fully Integrated or Best of Breed?

There are considerable benefits when an organization is working with a few solutions vendors as opposed to having many. There are many reasons that organizations have either gone with a primary EMR vendor or interfaced several applications to construct their EHR. Vendor selection is not a subject of this book. However, in order to maximize CPOE, the team must consider how the solutions store and move information across the departments and through the various venues of care.

For example, in most U.S. hospitals, the majority of patient admissions come through the Emergency Department (ED). Therefore, the ED team delivers care initially to the patient via triage, assessments and interventions that they document in their EMR or paper record. If the patient requires acute care admission, the ED physician makes a call to a colleague with admitting privileges. If the ED team uses an EMR, does all that data and information flow seamlessly into the inpatient EMR, or not? Do the orders from the ED flow or are they discontinued upon admission? How will you manage continuous life support orders across the platforms such as continuous IV drips (e.g. dopamine, a medicine to support the patient's blood pressure) or ventilators? Will the inpatient team be able to view the laboratory and vital sign results, or even the medication administration record?

Moreover, what advantage do you have with your vendors to solve complex issues as you proceed with CPOE? A single solution vendor will have a particular interest in working with you strategically to solve the issues above. While your best-of-breed vendors also desire to maintain your patronage, they may resort to pointing the finger at other vendors as problems arise. Therefore, you may need to commit additional time for design, build and test activities in a best-of-breed environment. In addition, one should not assume that single vendors have everything figured out for all the processes and scenarios you are automating.

The author has also seen many sites through the years where the hospital team suspends forward progress, as they look forward to the "new code" coming from their EMR vendor that will solve all their problems. Remember from the principles in Chap. 1 that new code is likely to bring new issues of its own. The author likes to remind colleagues that you should be careful for what you wish. In tribute to songwriter Stephen Stills, "If you can't be with the code you love, love the code you're with!"

4.1.3   Does the EMR Have a Physician-Friendly
Order Catalogue?

If you built your order catalogue from the beginning with CPOE in mind, then you are surely blessed and most likely in the minority. In the author's experience, many order catalogues began as departmental order tools that hospitals and systems later incorporated into their EMR. Hospitals developed many of these departmental order catalogues for the purpose of charge capture and accounting, rather than for ease of provider order entry.

Our favorite example is the electrocardiogram or ECG. Within a single hospital, multiple departments are capable of performing the test, and in fact, may have particular locations or times that they trade off performing the test. Prior to CPOE, hospitals often build multiple ECG orders to accommodate who would perform the ECG. Moreover, the persons performing the test would expect to get credit for the work on their departmental productivity. As a result, multiple ECG orders may exist in the order catalogue. In addition, the facility often develops complex business rules on who performs the ECG based on location, day of week, and/or time.

For example, there may be separate orders such as RN ECG (performed by nurse, credited to nursing productivity), ED ECG (performed by ED staff, credited to ED), CAR ECG (performed by cardiology technician and credited to that department), and RT ECG (performed by respiratory therapist and credited to that department). The business rules might sound like this: "The unit clerk, on the medical/surgical unit shall order a CAR ECG, Monday through Friday, from 8:00 AM until 4:30 PM. On nights and weekends, the unit clerk shall order an RT ECG, unless it is a stat study, at which time the clerk will order an RN ECG and the nurse will perform the study."

The situation, once CPOE is live, is that a physician needs a single order for ECG. It should never be the physician's responsibility to determine which department performs the test. The physician needs only to order the ECG. The hospital bears the burden to perform the ECG. The hospital's billing process should not be the responsibility of the physician.

There are many techniques to solving this issue and someone has to lead in this effort. A hospital might designate a single department to perform the ECG. The EMR team might create business rules that route the single ECG order to a common task list that all departments that perform ECGs might monitor. They may create business rules that route the singe ECG order electronically to the appropriate department who will then perform the ECG. On the other hand, they may choose to develop a manual process to rewrite all ECG orders and keep the unit clerk in charge. We would recommend the last alternative, however, to be a temporary work-around until the organization determines an electronic solution. However, in the case of the ECG, many departmental stakeholders may have passionate interests in maintaining the status quo, in protection of their charge credits for the test.

Similar to the ECG, the CPOE team should look at stress tests, echocardiograms, portable ultrasound (in obstetrics and for IV access), cardioversion (applying an electric shock to the heart, in the critical care unit versus in the operating suite), and temporary pacemakers. In the laboratory, similar problems arise in the case of simple tests like the CBC (complete blood count, the most frequent test in most U.S. hospitals) and the urinalysis (often the second most common test). We have found as many as 16 versions of CBC orders not to mention facilities that use the term Hemogram rather than CBC. We typically end up with three versions of the CBC for the physician's order catalogue: CBC with an automated differential count, CBC with no differential count, and CBC with a manual differential count.

Table 4.1 Comparison of two common chest x-rays

2-view chest x-ray	Portable chest x-ray
X-ray chest, 2 views	X-ray chest, 1 view
X-ray chest, PA and lateral	X-ray chest, AP
CXR	Portable CXR
Chest x-ray, PA/lat	Chest x-ray, AP

From these orders, the team can build business rules that cover the typical 16 types of CBC.[1]

A related issue is the concept of synonyms. Physicians have names and short hand designations for orders that they have used for years. This is particularly common among radiology imaging tests as Table 4.1 above demonstrates. The EMR will have a specific name for a study, such as a 2-view chest x-ray or a portable chest x-ray. Physicians have developed many alternative names through the years (and the unit clerk's have been good translators to order them by the EMR name).

At AHS, we used a two-symbol designation of the modality to begin each study. Thus, we used XR for x-ray, CT for computerized tomography, MR for magnetic resonance, US for ultrasound, and NM for nuclear medicine. We would follow this with the anatomic designation. Therefore, our example above would be XR chest 2 views and XR chest 1 view.

While one can teach such EMR designations to physicians, and they do adapt to them over time, they still want to search for orders the way they have handwritten them. Most EMR's allow you to create synonym orders, yet this may create confusion as well. Giving several names to the same order may lead to the physician pausing and second-guessing which test to choose from among similar choices.

In order to solve these issues, the CPOE team will need inter-disciplinary input from clinical and medical end-users, departmental stakeholders, and financial subject matter experts. It is important that you take the time to process these examples and develop solutions that work for the providers who order, the departments who fulfill the orders, and the persons who financially account for it. This topic represents a significant challenge the team faces as they evaluate their EMR in preparation for CPOE.

4.1.4   Does the EMR Have Medication Integration in Place?

The medication process is the foundation of CPOE. Regardless of which EMR you use, the twenty-first century CPOE project should have an integrated and seamless medication process. We would define this as follows:

---

[1] Based on initial CBC or differential counts, the lab may perform additional studies per policy. For example, if the automated differential count is abnormal, a business rule may trigger the process of having a hematology technician manually repeat the differential count. The technician's review may trigger the need for a full pathologist's review. The business rules and policy determine the correct intradepartmental workflow and billing.

1. The provider enters the medication order electronically with all five "medication rights" included as required fields. The ordering interface requires the provider to designate the right patient, right medication, right dose/strength/volume, right route, and the right frequency (i.e. at the right time). The order format allow the provider to indicate other order elements, such as stat (give it immediately), give with food, or not give if pulse less than 50 beats/min. All instructions relating to a single medication order should reside on that order, so that nurses and pharmacists would not have to look at multiple orders in reviewing one medication.

2. The instant the provider signs a medication order, the order becomes available to both the pharmacist (for verification) and the nurse (for review or acknowledgement) without any person manually re-entering the order.

3. If an unlicensed, non-provider enters the order (such as a medical student), the system does not process the order until which time a provider signs it.

4. If a licensed provider enters the order and reads it back to a provider, then the system forwards the order automatically to the provider for eventual electronic approval/signing.

5. Upon electronic ordering, the EMR includes a clinical decision support engine that allows the organization to create logic rules for error trapping (more on clinical decision support later[2]).

6. The pharmacist electronically reviews and verifies the electronic medication order, also benefiting from clinical decision support. The pharmacist's verification also releases any temporary holds that might occur if the facility has automated dispensing systems for their medications or on the electronic medication administration record (eMAR).

7. The nurse has an electronic process to acknowledge the presence of a new medication order.

8. The nurse has an electronic tool to see medication schedules and document administration. The nurse may also have access to a bar-code scanning system that double checks such elements as right medication for the right patient, and may log the administration date, time and/or person administering the medication.

9. The system captures the charges for the medication at some point during the process, dispensing or administration.

Systems may include other steps within the medication process. However, the medication process is the area of CPOE in which the organization can provide opportunities for both clinical decision support and a shorter time between the provider's decision to order and the fulfillment (i.e. administration of the medication) of that order, leading to better safety.

In modern day hospitals, the medication process may include robotic dispensing in the pharmacy, dispensing cabinets on the nursing units, and/or bar-code scanning systems to confirm that the nurse gives the right medication to the right patient at the right dose and time. Hospitals also improve the medication process by standardizing

---

[2] The author compares a CPOE system without clinical decision support to a car without brakes.

medication concentrations in intravenous (IV) fluids across the hospital or even health system. For example, a hospital might standardize insulin IV drips to deliver one unit of insulin per one milliliter (1 unit/1 mL) of fluid.

Hospitals may also limit their formulary to select one medication in a class of drugs (e.g. offer only one IV proton-pump inhibitor medication), rather than multiple agents which the clinicians may confuse. Hospitals should have a plan around medication safety and leverage CPOE within that plan. No one should rely on CPOE to solve medication safety issues. As stated in Chap. 1, one should not simply automate broken medication processes.

4.1.5 What Are the EMR Tools for Clinical Decision Support?

As the team designs and builds the CPOE platform, leadership should consider how CDS fits into the overall strategy. Each EMR vendor offers different tools to provide CDS integrated into the workflow, and this is especially important within the medication process. CDS comes in many forms. The goal is not to solve every care delivery problem when you implement CPOE, but rather to have a systematic approach. There is a fine balance between effective CDS and too much noise. The author has been guilty through the years of extremes at either end, as we work post implementation to fine-tune what the providers will accept and what yields results.

One should typically start a project with a plan on how much order set content he would provide to end-users. Through order sets, one can promote "suggested orders" for a diagnosis or condition, limit the doses and frequencies for medications and provide reminder statements of important interventions/considerations one should embrace or avoid. While these provide the physicians efficiency during order entry, they also begin to provide clinical guidance at the time of care.

Next, one provides links to the medical literature from within the order sets. While available in the workflow for the physician who desires more background, they should not impede the workflow with needless "pop-ups" or other barriers to the physician's efficiency.

Clinical alerting tools, on the other hand, should allow you to build specific decision alerts that do interrupt the workflow to address potential errors or harm. While EMR vendors do differ in their presentations, one should become familiar with how these tools works. Common reasons for alerts in the medication process include allergy-drug conflicts, drug duplications, dosing errors, drug-food interactions and disease specific alerts. The author will discuss his experiences with CDS in a later chapter. Excellent guides are available through HIMSS to assist organizations with CDS planning, governance, design and implementation.[3,4]

---

[3] Osheroff JA, editor. Improving medication use and outcomes with clinical decision support: a step-by-step guide. Chicago: Healthcare Information and Management Systems Society; 2009.

[4] HIMSS. Improving outcomes with clinical decision support: an implementer's guide. 2nd ed. Chicago: Healthcare Information and Management Systems Society; 2012.

4.1.6   Does the EMR Provide Electronic Documentation Tools for Providers?

As we discussed in Chap. 2, electronic documentation can provide additional efficiencies for the providers. As a health system or hospital rolls out CPOE, the leadership should make a conscious decision on what shall remain in the paper chart.

4.1.7   How Do Charges Drop Through Orders and Documentation?

In addition to the patient safety aspects of electronic orders, a hospital is very interested in using the EMR to capture accurate and timely charges. Regarding medication orders, CPOE allows the hospital to charge upon the nurse's administration of the medication rather than when the pharmacy or med cabinet dispenses it. Prior to CPOE, many hospitals are dropping charges on administration on their inpatient units, but not in the ED or the Surgical Department. Therefore, the team will need to look at each patient care area and determine the proper workflow and charging once CPOE goes live.

The project team should look at billable supplies as well. CPOE may allow the facility to tie charges to orders and clinical documentation, and no longer require the nursing team to document charges through a different mechanism. Typically, a hospital should be able to improve charge accuracy once CPOE is live.

4.1.8   Is There a Content Process for Order Sets and Documentation?

As the author discussed earlier, the CPOE team project should include a clear process for order set design and maintenance. Likewise, the team should create a mechanism for providing solutions and maintenance in the area of provider documentation. The more providers document electronically, the more they will be expecting enhancements and opportunities to improve their efficiency. The hospital will only create ill will if they do not have a plan in place to maintain this content and offer quick turnaround of appropriate enhancement requests.

4.1.9   How Do Providers Maintain Problem Lists?

Modern day EMR's will have some mechanism for providers to enter and update a list of problems for the patient. As he discussed in Chap. 2, the author recommends that the physicians should own the Problem List. Therefore, the team should determine how the providers might accomplish this within their workflow. In addition, the Problem List should be visible to the provider when he orders, he documents, and when he makes key medical decisions. Moreover, the EMR should leverage the Problem List as a tool for handoffs and clinical decision support.

At the time of this book, the Office of the National Coordinator (ONC) has recommended that SNOMED[5] be the code set that providers will utilize to document Problem Lists in compliance with the Stage 2 "Meaningful Use" provisions under HITECH.[6] Therefore, the EMR should have SNOMED CT available to the providers for the entry and update of the Problem List. EMR's may also permit the providers to enter "diagnoses" using the latest version of ICD-x.[7] In addition, there may be the ability to tag problems that the provider is actively addressing during a hospital encounter as well as those he is not addressing.

The CPOE plan should include how the providers will leverage the Problem List in the care of individual patients. The author recommends that the Problem List provide useful context for medical decision-making. Therefore, the providers should be able to see the list of Problems when placing orders, as well as documenting care and treatment plans at admission (within the History and Physical, or H & P), daily rounds (within daily Progress Notes) and at discharge (with the Discharge Summary). For example, the physician should clearly note at the time of admission if the patient has chronic illness such as COPD (chronic obstructive pulmonary disease) or diabetes mellitus. In addition, by noting the problems in the Progress Notes and the H & P, the provider uses them to communicate co-morbidities to any covering provider as well as to the rest of the patient care team. The author has seen schemes in which nurses update and maintain the Problem List instead of physicians. This typically leads to a Problem List that is either too general (diabetes, rather than diabetes with ophthalmic complications) or too superfluous (constipation, or prone to fall). The one exception one tends to make is to include chronic infections that require isolation, such as MRSA (methicillin-resistent *Staph. aureus*) and *C. difficile* colonization, which the infection practitioner adds to the Problem List for longitudinal consideration for the safety of patients.

4.1.10 How Will Providers Co-sign Verbal and Telephone CPOE Orders?

Even with CPOE, the providers will give a percentage of verbal/telephone orders. The team will need to ensure that the EMR routes these orders and that the providers

[5] SNOMED CT (Systematized Nomenclature of Medicine--Clinical Terms) is a comprehensive clinical terminology, originally created by the College of American Pathologists (CAP) and, as of April 2007, owned, maintained, and distributed by the International Health Terminology Standards Development Organisation (IHTSDO), a not-for-profit association in Denmark. http://www.nlm.nih.gov/research/umls/Snomed/snomed_main.html.

[6] The Health Information Technology for Economic and Clinical Health (HITECH) Act, enacted as part of the American Recovery and Reinvestment Act of 2009 (i.e. the "stimulus" plan of 2009).

[7] International Classification of Diseases, World Health Organization. Currently the U.S. uses ICD-9, with plans to implement ICD-10 in late 2014 and ICD-11 in 2015.

sign them in a timely manner. Many EMR's provide some type of Inbox for this function. However, the providers will refuse to sign a small number of these orders for a variety of reasons (wrong physician, wrong order, or wrong patient). The team will need to determine a process for providers to refuse to sign such orders and determine how the EMR will reroute these orders for completion.

4.1.11   Testing of the CPOE System

The Project Manager needs to ensure that the teams thoroughly test and validate all aspects of the CPOE system. The team should perform unit testing of all orders, including medications and order sentences. The team may want to audit the current production system for orders and order sentences that providers utilize on paper, to ensure that the system can properly support the historical ordering processes. The team should also plan to build additional order sentences once the system goes live.

The team should complete functional and integration testing to ensure that all aspects of major ordering processes work without error. This is especially important with the medication process, which includes the physician's order, nurse review, pharmacist's verification, nurse's administration, and charge capture. Testing should also allow the team to evaluate the CDS in the system.

In addition, the author recommends that the pilot unit/hospital perform parallel testing with both a patient scenario, then with several real patients. By this, we mean that several end-users replicate their ordering and documentation processes in the CPOE environment prior to activation. This will help the end-users to evaluate the workflow and ascertain if the system has all elements that they need for patient care. We do recommend that the parallel testing not include the patient's actual name or PHI (protected health information).

4.1.12   Critical Success Factors for CPOE Pilot(s)

Assuming that the project will have some type of CPOE pilot, the team should determine what pilot success would look like. The following points should serve as a compass for physician automation and CPOE activities. The author will discuss these areas more in Chap. 5.

- Clear Vision: Everyone should know why they are automating physician workflow and be able to articulate a clear description of what they expect to achieve and how end-users will achieve it.
- Defined Clinical, Operational, and Financial Goals: Each goal must be clearly defined and measureable, and align with the organization's vision. The team should collect appropriate benchmark data prior to implementing CPOE, against which they will measure improvements.

- Leadership: Executive and clinical leadership must have tenacity, be visible, and vocal – constantly reinforcing and communicating the vision and goals. It is critical to involve as many physicians, nurses, unit clerks, pharmacists, and other end-users as possible in the process of planning and change, and have a critical mass of committed champions and super-users. Automating physician workflow must be a primary focus of the organization during the process.
- Value Proposition: Each end-user must internalize the vision and goals to the point that each can answer the question: "What's in it for me, and for my patient(s)?" While organizational wins are important, success depends on the individuals who perceive value and can personalize and internalize the value.
- Well-defined Learning and Education Plans: Training should be scenario-driven rather than functionality-driven to stress how workflow will occur with physician automation and CPOE. They should offer different venues for training including web-based learning to accommodate various learning styles. The leadership must stress best practices at every opportunity.
- Device Access: Each end-user shall have ready access to a device when and where they need it. The technical infrastructure will be reliable and with excellent response times.
- Culture: Project will assess culture of the organization early in the process, determining the values, beliefs and behaviors of the leadership, medical staff, and end-users. The team will check the "pulse" of the organization regularly to ensure that communication and end-user engagement is successful.
- Process Optimization: Process redesign will involve multidisciplinary end-users to identify current inefficiencies and seek to optimize the new processes, rather than use to automate them. One should seek to leverage the technology to optimize the end-user experience around safety, quality and efficiency, rather than automate existing processes.
- Measure: Project metrics will establish baselines, and then quantify the clinical, operational, and financial benefits of the project. The team should revisit processes that do not achieve the predicted benefits to understand why, and investigate modifications for the future.

4.2 Key Points

- The Project Manager should have a written project plan that documents the timeline and resources to support the CPOE project scope.
- The project team should fully understand the current hospital automation including systems in place and amount of integration across systems.
- The team must address many clinical and physician processes for successful implementation of CPOE.
- The leadership must determine its strategy for piloting CPOE.

- The Project Manager must develop a plan for testing the system prior to pilot,
- There are known critical success factors that the team may address prior to their CPOE pilot.

4.3   Fingernails on the Chalkboard

- **There is no project plan**
  There are a large number of decisions and steps involved in a CPOE project. Each project task should clearly document the responsible person, resources and a timeline for completion.
- **"We are only doing partial CPOE."**
  We would define "partial CPOE" as only requiring providers to enter certain orders electronically and leaving the rest as handwritten orders. This creates inefficient workflow for both the physicians and the nurses, and may result in end-users who miss critical orders. In addition, it is hard for the leadership to promote CPOE as a patient safety initiative when it is fragmented.
- **Doing CPOE without an integrated medication process**
  With one study suggesting an increase in mortality from a fragmented medication process, hospitals should not pursue CPOE without a seamlessly integrated electronic process.

Chapter 5
Change Management

Abstract The author discusses the importance of a structured change management methodology and lays out specific roles and responsibilities for a successful CPOE engagement. This chapter presents specific steps and communication that the author has successfully used for the past 12 years in deploying CPOE. He also introduces the concept of the CPOE Change Readiness Assessment that assesses the organization and begins the leadership's preparation for a successful CPOE project.

> *It is always easier to talk about change than to make it*
> *– Alvin Toffler, futurist*

While many healthcare leaders see CPOE as a daunting challenge, the author likes to see it as the best opportunity an organization has at developing great structure and skills in change management. One should start with a strong foundation of the field. The author gives his highest recommendation to *Leading Change*[1] by John P. Kotter, as the must read book for all healthcare leaders on the science and practicality of change management. In order to succeed with a CPOE implementation, one must first acknowledge that you need to manage change. Then you must act on that knowledge and put a proper change management plan into place. While vision and executive leadership are foundational requirements for successful CPOE projects, failing to define and execute your change management plan will make it extremely difficult to succeed at your efforts.

While there are many definitions for change management, the author recommends the following: "The process, tools and techniques to manage the people-side of change to achieve the required business results." One should discriminate this from the concept of "change control", which the author would define as: "The process, tools and techniques to manage the technology-side of change to achieve the required business results." In lay terms, change management is leading people through a change initiative. Change control is really the discipline an organization uses to thoughtfully evaluate, manage, approve, implement and track changes in their technology platform in order to support their business processes. The author often sees the terms used interchangeably, but in fact, they are quite distinct. There

---

[1] Kotter JP. Leading change. Boston: Harvard Business Review Press; 1996.

P.A. Smith, *Making Computerized Provider Order Entry Work*,
Health Information Technology Standards,
DOI 10.1007/978-1-4471-4243-0_5, © Springer-Verlag London 2013

is real danger if you are executing your change management plan and your technology team thinks you are talking about change control. Both are critical for success. This chapter outlines steps and tools we have refined over the past 10 years for CPOE projects. Each project's plan varies based on the schedule, resources, size and objectives of the organization.

Change management is critical to a CPOE implementation for several reasons. First, one must consider a phrase the author first coined over a decade ago to an executive team: "Everything in a hospital begins with a physician order. Therefore, when you change the way a physician orders, you change almost every process in the hospital." So this statement holds true whether you are converting from paper to electronic, from printed orders to electronic, or even if you are changing from one CPOE platform to another. Once a provider initiates orders electronically, CPOE affects how the downstream users receive, interpret, and fulfill each order. Consequentially, many former processes will no longer be relevant to the new CPOE processes. Moreover, you would like to go beyond simply automating the former paper process. Instead, one's goal is to transform the ordering process in order to obtain a more efficient and effective workflow for improved outcomes and safer patient care.

We have all seen projects in which we have not successfully managed change. We may have started out with great expectations for an initiative only to find later that we have lowered productivity. While we are always on the lookout for those persons actively resisting CPOE, we also may experience end-users acting out with various forms of passive resistance. When we do not successfully manage change, our end-users may exhibit some common signs and symptoms, such as:

- Arguing about the need to change
- Calling in sick during training or around implementation
- Not showing up for training (physically or mentally)
- Refusing to fully adopt new workflows and/or developing work-around processes
- Reverting to their old way of doing things
- Creating "us versus them" divisions
- Threatening to resign, or resigning
- Threats or making external claims to regulatory groups
- Focusing on risks and ignoring potential rewards
- Not achieving the potential outcomes/benefits
- Cancelling the initiative altogether

As the author previously noted, the hospital unit clerk/secretary (HUC), in the pre-CPOE world, often spends a considerable amount of time faxing or transmitting medication orders to the hospital pharmacy. In addition, this role may enter the majority of the non-medication orders in the pre-CPOE hospital. In the CPOE environment, this function of the HUC disappears and that role no longer participates in the medication ordering process since the physician directly enters the medication order and it immediately appears to the pharmacist for order verification. Since the HUC's prior workflow, tasks and competencies are no longer valid, it is important that the CPOE team help the organization redesign workflow and accountabilities around a new paradigm. Moreover, the HUC's manager must clearly articulate how he plans to change, rather than eliminate, the HUC's role. Failure on the part of the manager to communicate the process will likely create a "stakeholder" who may fear job elimination and create dissonance about CPOE to everyone with his circle of influence (especially the doctors and nurses). These conversations, however, must be two-way dialogues, not simply the manager telling the HUC "This is the way it is going to be." In the example of the HUC, many organizations redefine the role around customer (patient and patient's family) service in addition to communication on the nursing unit.

The change management plan begins by assessing the culture and climate of the organization with the final aim of organization readiness for a successful implementation. The plan should consist of several key phases during the CPOE project and function independent and parallel to the technology design, build, test, and activation steps. The author recommends that the initial phase be a CPOE readiness (or change readiness) assessment. The team uses this assessment to plan the specific steps for organizational readiness. The change management plan should integrate with the project plan and have several defined components that exist in every project:

- Stakeholder Engagement
- Communication
- Training
- Workflow
- Performance Management
- Employee Impact and Retention
- Knowledge Management
- Executive and Leadership Coaching
- Patient/Community Engagement
- Physician Engagement

Each of these areas should have a defined scope, tools and a responsible leader who the organization will hold accountable. The change manager and the project manager integrate project/change tasks into the unified project plan so that transparency occurs. In a large health system, the change manager has more face-time with the hospital leadership than the project manager does. In a single hospital implementation, both are readily available and visible to both the facility and project leaders. Once again, it is important to note that the project manager has overall project responsibility and ensures that the technology readiness occurs, while the change manager focuses on the readiness of the people.

The author recommends that you not have classic IT resources lead the change management efforts, but rather have the change manager educating the IT team on the roles, responsibilities and key processes of the change management engagement. If you do not have an experienced change manager, you can find candidates with background in healthcare management, organizational behavior or industrial psychology. Regardless of education, the ideal change manager must be organized, confident, flexible, and collaborative in addition to superb presentation and people skills. The change manager must be able to facilitate honest dialogue from the Boardroom all the way down to the end-users. While the manager starts each engagement with a defined plan, she must be able to remain flexible and consultative, adapting as necessary to overcome resistance and obtain buy-in.

5.1 Key Events of the Change Management Plan

In this chapter, The author will discuss the key change management events one should consider for a CPOE project. In Chap. 6, he will provide additional granularity for those readers who want more detail. In the single hospital setting, the change manager may take on one of the champion roles. In the multi-hospital setting, the change manager focuses on knowledge transfer to the project champions, coaching and accountability. Because organizational culture is such a strong determinant of project success, the change manager focuses more on the objectives of the project rather than the specific techniques or tasks. One is humbled quickly if you think that you have a rigid engagement plan for change. The author has seen that even in a three-hospital system, cultures vary from hospital to hospital. So one should keep in mind, "If you have seen one CPOE implementation, you have seen one CPOE implementation."[2]

5.2 CPOE Change Readiness Assessment

Prior to having a formal CPOE Kick-off at a facility, it is beneficial that you complete a CPOE Change Readiness Assessment (CRA). The CRA phase is typically a 90-day period and includes an initial workshop, leadership interviews, a formal cultural assessment, and additional change management activities. These activities include a communication assessment, learning assessment, stakeholder analysis, and employee retention assessment. These efforts will assist the site and CPOE Steering Committee to determine an appropriate CPOE activation date.

As we mentioned above, the cultures of hospitals are unique, so it is important that you have a rigorous process of assessments to understand where you are starting. Each hospital/organization faces change uniquely, based on experiences, availability of resources, and competing priorities. CPOE has major impact on workflow throughout the organization and represents a major change initiative for employees, physicians and patients.

Once you understand the culture and climate of each facility, your specific approach to achieving your objectives will adjust throughout your project. The CRA is critical, as it allows the change manger to understand the specific strengths of the

---

[2] The author has found this to be an important reminder to the team as they complete their first CPOE implementation.

leadership team and the opportunities to address gaps that may present challenges to success. Through the years, the author has evaluated many CPOE projects in the industry and identified common risks that impede the success of those initiatives: lack of baseline data, unidentified risks that surface and jeopardize the project, ineffective change interventions not aligned with the actual organizational needs and risks, and employees and physicians disengaged from the process. The author has designed and refined the CRA to address these unnecessary CPOE project risks.

The change manager, through the CRA, assesses the organization's current ability to manage the change of CPOE. Activities include the identification of major risks, competing priorities, change enablers and barriers, as well as the development and execution of key strategies, action plans and interventions to facilitate effective change. One should ask key questions of the organization in this process:

- What other projects/initiatives is the organization planning during the CPOE project timeline?
- How is the hospital performing clinically, financially, and operationally?
- What are the key business challenges that the hospital is facing?
- Is there a business case for CPOE at this time?
- What examples of major change has the facility faced in the past 5 years? Were they successful or not?

The organization benefits as the CRA provides benchmark operational and cultural data, identifies risks and competing priorities and allows for a focused engagement and communication plan for CPOE. Through the years, the author has utilized various tools and key events during the CRA, and is always challenging him and his teams to improve them. However, each step in the CRA has a specific intent and contributes to the overall project success. The author describes these tools in further detail below.

5.3 Executive Preparation Call

The executive sponsor of the CPOE project and the change manager should hold an initial call with the executive team to lay the groundwork for a successful CPOE engagement. The executive sponsor lays out the 40,000-ft view of the CPOE timeline and the importance of the CRA. It is important that the executive sponsor lead this call in order to introduce and promote the change manager to the facility executives.

An important concept is that the change manager may initially have little influence or relationship with the executive team. This is the first example of "specific intent." The executive sponsor introduces the change manager and promotes the importance of this person and the process to create empowerment at the highest level of the facility.

The main outcome of the executive sponsor is to secure the commitment of the executive team to work with the change manager to find 2 upcoming days in which every executive is available for the CRA workshop and interviews. Thereafter, the change manager typically works with the executive assistant to indentify the date and schedule the attendees, for not only the workshop, but also the individual interviews.

5.4   Executive CRA Workshop

The CPOE leadership team[3] presents the 4-h Executive CRA Workshop at the facility with the entire facility executive team[4] in attendance. In addition, the facility invites most directors as well as personnel with key responsibilities for CPOE:

- Medical staff leadership
- Clinical informatics lead
- Pharmacy director
- Human Resources director
- Clinical nursing directors such as Critical Care and Emergency Department
- Surgery manager or director
- Patient Financial Services and/or Registration director
- Health Information Management (HIM) director
- Information Technology director
- Physician liaison (person/personnel providing physician "elbow support")

The project leadership team's specific intent of the workshop is directly observing the facility's team dynamics: do they participate, do they collaborate, do they speak their minds, and do they have fun? Moreover, it is important to remember that the facility participants are also evaluating the project team during this initial event: do they know what they are doing, will they guide us through these difficult waters, and can they be trusted?

The CPOE team provides an overview of the CPOE project. Activities include identifying the specific facility CPOE Champions in addition to physician engagement strategies. The author discusses the specific CPOE Champions in detail later in this chapter. Chapter 6 provides a detailed agenda for the CRA.

5.5   Leadership Interviews

Members of the CPOE team conduct the leadership interviews the afternoon and morning after the workshop. The interviewers, working in pairs, spend approximately 45 min with each individual who attended the CRA workshop. These interviews determine competing priorities, attitudes towards CPOE, and the commitment of the executive team, leadership, and medical staff for moving forward with CPOE.

---

[3] Typically, this team includes the Executive Sponsor, the Medical Director, Clinical Applications Director, IT Director, Informatics Lead and the Change Manager.

[4] The team schedules the event so that every member of the C-Suite (CEO, COO, CFO, CNO and CMO) attends. We recommend you not hold the event otherwise.

These interviews also help to identify fears and concerns in regards to CPOE as well as the views of how leadership and executives will respond to resistance by staff and/or physicians. While the interviews help the team to identify key opportunities and provide useful insights, the specific comments are strictly confidential.

After a brief introduction and review of the process, one can typically use questions like the ones below. If you already know of a specific competing priority or conflict, you may also address that during these interviews.

1. Please share some background on your career and your time here?
2. Are there any added responsibilities that are not apparent in your title?
3. What do you see as your role in this project?
4. What do you think we will gain by doing this project?
5. What are your biggest fears about the project?
6. Is there anything going on at the facility that would be a competing interest (e.g. upcoming accreditation survey, renovations, or new service line launch)?
7. Do you have any personnel and/or resource concerns?
8. Do you perceive any obstacles to the successful implementation of CPOE?
9. Please name one broken process that you feel may be exposed with CPOE, and why?
10. How to you think the CEO will deal with resistant physicians? In addition, for the CEO: How do you think you will deal with resistant physicians?
11. What is your preferred method of contact: phone, email, or working through an assistant?
12. Is there anything else you wish to discuss, related to this project?

For the C-Suite/Executives only:

13. Is your leadership prepared for any downturn in revenue of volumes during the transition to CPOE?
14. Have you prepared for any reduction in personal efficiency during the transition to CPOE?
15. How do see yourself dealing with resistant physicians?

The specific intent of these interviews is for the CPOE team to understand not only the answers to the questions, but the transparency of the individuals in answering them, and the consistency across the leadership team. It is also to build rapport with each other for the challenges ahead.

5.6 Organizational Culture Survey

About 1 week after the Executive CRA Workshop and interviews, we have the CEO personally send an email to each member of the management team[5] to complete a confidential online survey of organizational culture. The team should provide the

---

[5] Management team typically consists of the managers and above at the hospital.

CEO with a cover letter to the management team, with a short mention of the upcoming CPOE project, the importance of culture, and the fact that this is a confidential third-party survey of their culture. The author recommends the CEO open the survey for only a week to develop a sense of urgency and typically, most of the management team respond. For the past decade, he has used Denison Consulting for this process,[6] specifically, *The Denison Survey of Organizational Culture.* This 10-min, online survey measures 12 aspects of the facility's culture. The author specifically leverages the results to assess areas of strength at each facility, as well as areas that will need additional focus to ensure successful CPOE implementation. The CPOE team reviews the survey in conjunction with the results of the leadership interviews and their observation of team dynamics. The author discusses *The Denison Survey of Organizational Culture* in more detail in Chap. 6.

5.7   Leadership Workshop

Once they receive the results of the *Denison Survey of Organizational Culture*, the CPOE leadership team jointly reviews the results, and correlates them to the interviews and direct observations. They should focus their assessment on elements of the culture that are consistent across all three components (survey, interviews and direct observation). With this information in mind, they then conduct a CPOE Leadership Workshop, approximately a month after the initial CRA Workshop, as the second hour of a 2-h management team meeting. This workshop provides the facility's management team with a brief overview of CPOE and the list of the facility Champions for the project. In addition, it is an opportunity for the CPOE team to validate the results of their Denison Survey and the CRA to date. The author specifically likes the participants to sit in a U-shape or circle and have one team member facilitate the presentation and discussion. The team's specific intent includes understanding the management team dynamics, answering their questions on the CPOE project, and validating their cultural assessment findings.

The CPOE team should meet with the executives just prior to the event. They do a brief run-through of the Denison survey at a high level and discuss their key objectives for validation with the management team at the upcoming workshop. They often have one or two findings from the Denison that they wish to probe more deeply, and they ask for the executive's permission to do so with their managers and directors.

The CPOE team have previously asked the executive team to hold their normal management team meeting (up to 1 h) so that they can observe format, style and team dynamics during this event as well. They also ask the executive team to listen and watch their hospital leadership team as the CPOE team presents the Denison survey results during the workshop, and the management team responds actively during the event.

---

[6] www.DenisonConsulting.com.

The author observes that he repeatedly gets feedback that "it is rare for anyone to give them specific feedback on any survey." This event specifically allows the CPOE team to confirm the results of the CRA, based on the management team's feedback and their observations during the meeting. Often the CPOE team will hold a quick debrief with the executives to elicit their observations from the workshop.

5.8 Change Manager Activities

During the CRA phase, the change manager personally meets with each of the facility CPOE Champions to explain specific roles and responsibility, review tasks and due dates on the project timeline, and obtain formal review and sign-off on a Knowledge Transfer Agreement (See Appendix B). The Knowledge Transfer Agreement not only serves as documentation, but also is an effective accountability tool. In cases where the CPOE Champion is not an executive, the change manager also obtains the executive's sign-off on the form.

The change manager works with the Executive Sponsor and schedules a recurring monthly CPOE champions meeting on the executive calendar. All executives, the CPOE champions, the project manager, engagement leaders, and key members of the CPOE team (IT leader, informatics leader, etc.) commit to this monthly meeting. The change manager drives the agenda, starts each meeting with a recap of the accomplishments of the past 30 days. Then the Champions and other key members each give an update on their areas of accountability for the project. The format is consistent for each report: accomplishments of the past 30 days including data to support their processes, and ending each report with the plans for the next 30 days.[7] The project manager reviews the status of the project and the key project milestones chart reminding the team of achievements and the journey ahead. The champions should have addressed any project risks and mitigations during their respective monthly reports. After a time for open discussion, the change manager reviews the "next 30 days," specifying key milestones, events, deliverables and dates. The author has seen great results keeping everyone focused on only 30-day periods of time.

The change manager also completes the following deliverables during the remaining weeks of the CRA.

5.9 Communication Assessment

The change manager completes a communication assessment with the facility's CPOE Communication Champion. This assessment identifies the communication tools and methods used within the facility, as well as areas that may need

---

[7] This format supports that CPOE is a complex change initiative and we tackle it as if we were eating an elephant, "one bite at a time!"

improvement to ensure successful communication of CPOE. The communication team utilizes the assessment to develop a plan. They engage the facility and medical staff and inform them of the changes associated with the CPOE implementation. This plan helps minimize rumors, confusion, surprises, resistance, and misinformation that may arise during implementation.

The communication team also leads the development of a theme for the facility's project. The themes that the staff finds most popular are usually those that encourage the executive team to appear in costume. These create great memories for the facility, from kick-off to go live.

5.10 Learning Assessment

The change manager meets with the facility CPOE Training Champion to identify the facility's current training format, resources, and success with previous training. The team records the number of classrooms and the capacity of each room. They use this learning assessment to develop a training plan for outlining the course materials, class format, and time schedules for each end-user group requiring training for CPOE.

5.11 Stakeholder Analysis

The facility's CPOE Stakeholder Identification & Engagement Champion conduct a stakeholder analysis to identify key roles, groups and individuals, their power and influence within the facility, and their current and desired levels of commitment. With this assessment information, they develop a stakeholder engagement plan. They identify effective strategies to engage key stakeholders and achieve desired levels of commitment to the CPOE project.

5.12 Retention Assessment

The change manager helps the facility CPOE Employee Impact & Retention Champion complete a retention assessment to identify key facility CPOE team members who are critical to project success. The Champion reviews individuals based on the years of employment at the facility, as well as their internal and external drivers. The goal is to create incentives for individuals to stay with the project through its conclusion. The champion uses this assessment to create a retention plan to ensure the key individuals remain engaged and committed to the project through implementation.

The change manager also obtains the organizational chart and chain of command structure from the Employee Impact Champion. They also begin to compile job descriptions which the facility may need to modify prior to CPOE activation.

5.13   Key Roles and Project Champions

There are key roles that one must include in every project. The author has discussed the design, build, and test teams in Chap. 4. They are responsible for the technology that we will implement in the CPOE project. You should also have an implementation team. They are responsible for the activation events that result in a successful go live of the system and the immediate support of the end-users. In a single hospital, these teams may consist in the same individuals and typically work within the IT department. On the other hand, they may be consultants, which you bring in specifically for your CPOE project. Though some organizations may have mature change management departments within their operations, the author has found that many do not have a defined process or infrastructure to tackle a CPOE project. In fact, he commonly finds in healthcare that leaders, and maybe even some project managers, have only a small picture of change management. "Oh, you mean training," or "We already have a theme for our project," are typical warning signs that you may not be on the right track for successfully managing the change of your CPOE project.

You should also have designated informatics and IT support staff at each facility. These staff members should remain responsible for day-to-day support of your end-users. You should not give them change management leadership roles. This is a rule to which the author has occasionally made exception, and it has all but once turned out to be a bad decision. There are two reasons for this. First, the end-users see them as IT support and it shifts the CPOE project emphasis in their minds from being an organizational transformation project to being an IT implementation project. Secondly, as the CPOE activation draws near, they have unlimited tasks to accomplish such as ensuring physicians are attending training, answering questions, granting remote access, and proctoring training classes. The one exception in the past decade was indeed an exceptional person who had influence and power in the organization beyond her title. As brilliant and exceptional as you see your own people, the author recommends you heed this advice and not play the odds.

The other requirement he makes is to make sure each champion has the right level of position, influence and power in the organization to accomplish the tasks in each role. These champions are responsible for activities across departments and at various levels throughout the organization. The one exception is the Knowledge Management Champion. This person maintains the online facility repository of all documents and calendars for the project. Most facilities already have a designated person in such a role. In most other cases, you will want to select a vice president or director (i.e. positions above manager) for each non-physician role and not select someone who only has influence in one department. As he discusses each champion below, he will offer some common suggestions for each role. These summaries may be helpful as you identify your champions and assign them their goals for each role (also see summaries in Appendix A).

5.14 Stakeholder Engagement

The Stakeholder Engagement Champion identifies major constituencies within the organization and their major issues. The champion assesses each group's current and desired levels of commitment. He then designs and executes strategies to effectively engage them to achieve desired levels of commitment for the CPOE project. The champion may identify key individuals within each group who are leaders/ influencers within that group, as well as those who otherwise pose risk to project success. The ultimate goals of this champion are to identify the key stakeholder groups and best understand and address their issues and needs through the transition to CPOE.

Following the four principles in Sect. 1.1, this champion is responsible for the "what" and the "whom" in the second principle, "What's in it for me?" From this assessment, the champion can collaborate with the Communication Champion to determine and deliver the correct answer to each group. The Stakeholder Engagement Champion finds and documents answers to the following key questions:

- Who are the major stakeholder groups whom CPOE impacts and how?
- How significant is the change that they will experience during the CPOE project?
- How will the organization ensure engagement of the stakeholders for buy-in of the change?
- How do the various stakeholders view the change?
- What sub-cultures exist, and how do they affect the interactions across the various groups?
- Is the facility's climate and culture fully supportive of CPOE, and if not, what specific concerns do each group have?
- Are there any old processes that stakeholders will find hard to let go?
- Are end-users engaged in finding opportunities to leverage CPOE processes and gain ownership of the change?

The Stakeholder Champion owns the following deliverables:

- Identify Stakeholder Groups and describe the attributes that make them a significant group
- Assess current and desired commitment levels of each group
- Determine and assess leaders/influencers for each group
- Collaborate with the Communication Champion to develop effective strategies to deliver the key messages to achieve the group's commitment to project success

- Facilitate meetings with each group to share project goals, their involvement and, through active interchange, determine how CPOE will affect them and provide opportunities for gain.
- Educate leadership to reinforce the importance of effective stakeholder engagement.

The Champion must understand the organization and not show favoritism toward any one group. Commonly, the facility selects a vice president (member of the executive team) for this role. The Champion pulls together ad hoc groups early in the process to ensure proper identification of key stakeholder groups.

Key benefits of this process include:

- Identify risks, barriers and enablers of change for each stakeholder group
- Develop ownership within each group for successful change
- Improve the ability to promote buy-in
- Identify and manage resistance
- Align facility leadership to the needs and concerns of the groups
- Achieve effective communication during the project
- Avoid unnecessary conflicts that may undermine the project
- Promote collaboration across the groups to address and solve potential problems

The work of the Stakeholder Engagement Champion enables more effective change management. The following risks might occur if you choose to skip this process:

- Individuals or groups may become unengaged, disenfranchised, or even hostile to the project
- These groups drown out the intended project message with "hearsay, rumor, and innuendo"
- The leadership fails to align with the needs and concerns of the groups as the "What's in it for me?" question remains unanswered
- Poor decision-making, poor buy-in and/or poor morale
- Individuals or groups start acting out and compromising the project success
- Behavior and attitudes become inconsistent and detrimental to the CPOE initiative

The major time commitments for this champion occur during the CRA as the initial stakeholder identification occurs and during the first week or two, starting at the facility's CPOE kick-off event. The latter time includes some specific focus groups to begin the engagement process. Since the author has mentioned the hospital unit clerks (HUCs) as a specific stakeholder group, he will share the specific engagement process that has worked for multiple CPOE projects:

The HUCs are a particularly high-risk stakeholder group as they have one of the greatest job impacts from a CPOE project. In the non-CPOE world, they are the gatekeeper of the order processes as physicians write orders, and the HUCs either transcribes the order onto paper MARs (medication administration records), into electronic order systems, or transmits them (as often is in the case of medications to the pharmacist). CPOE ideally removes the HUC completely from this medication process, eliminating 40–60 % of their workflow. So, it is natural that the major question running through the head of the HUC is, "When will my job be eliminated?" This naturally leads to fear and resistance. The team needs to address this at the start of the project. The change manager facilitates the initial meeting of the HUCs as a demonstration to the Stakeholder Champion. The author recommends that the Champion contact the manager/director over the HUCs during the CRA and schedule a mandatory meeting of all HUCs, including day and night shift employees. The ideal day for the meeting is the day of the facility's CPOE kick-off, or a day or two before this event. Any delays beyond the kick-off will lead to the HUCs' resistance.

The meeting should be in a room that you arrange in a collaborative seating arrangement, such as a U-shape or semi-circle with tables on which they can make notes. The facilitator stands at the front with a blank flip chart or white board, and no projector. The Stakeholder Champion sits in a position in which he can watch the participants and they can watch him. The champion should be open in body language and appear interested in the process with paper for notes (and no opportunity for checking email). The manager of the HUCs should also attend, but not actively participate or dominate the process.

The change manager starts with a brief introduction of herself and the purpose of the meeting. She specifically gives a brief explanation that, "The facility is kicking off a project called CPOE or computerized provider order entry. This means that physicians will no longer be writing their orders on paper, but entering them directly into the computer. How do you think that will impact your job here?"

The facilitator allows the group to dialogue on this question, and comments will usually arise around how it will affect their job, and eventually someone will verbalize the potential for job elimination, such as "I should start looking for a job" or "They won't be needing me anymore?" It is important now to be patient and allow them to get the issue on the table before the facilitator proceeds with the exercise.

The facilitator then proceeds with, "Most hospitals find that CPOE will free up about 40-60 % of your current workday, and we are here to get your ideas on how we can better utilize that time on your unit. So let's start by me writing down up here that we are no longer entering orders or sending orders to the pharmacy" (at which time she writes down entering orders and sending orders at the top of the flipchart/board and intentionally puts an X through each). "Now typically, there are other things that you do in you day, that often take a "back seat" to the orders. Please help me list those out so that we can all understand them." At this point, the facilitator is making a list of at least 16 and typically 18 other things that the HUCs do at the hospital. The facilitator will take each one down, asks questions on most to better understand and record each process, and tries to engage as many in the group as possible in the exercise. As the list grows, it quickly dwarfs the two items at the top. If they don't include it, the facilitator will usually add, "Don't forget the doctors may come to you for help as you are the current experts on entering orders and what we call things around here."

The comes the critical question, "Of all these things we have listed, which do you see as the most valuable for our mission to take care of our patients?" The facilitator will then help them rank the top three. The facilitator should then step back and admire the list with the HUCs. The ultimate goal is to help them clearly see their contribution to their unit, the patients, nurses and doctors that they work with each day. The facilitator gives them plenty of time to understand the message and communicate next steps as their manager and the Stakeholder Champion will meet with them in the subsequent weeks to help define their new roles and responsibilities once CPOE is live. Obviously, it is critical that the manager follows through on redesigning the roles and responsibilities as well as the resultant job description. The Stakeholder Champion tracks the progress and reports at the monthly Champion updates. These activities succeed in overcoming fear among end-users, and serve to create an environment of accountability for this aspect of the project.

The Stakeholder Champion also leverages other project events to engage the various stakeholder groups, such as workflow sessions as well as specific physician meetings (anesthesia and ED providers), which a physician will facilitate, rather than the champion. In addition, the champion collaborates with the Communication Champion to make sure that the Communication Plan address successful communication to each stakeholder group.

5.15 Communication

The Communication Champion owns the overall Communication Plan for the CPOE project. This champion's objective is that they engage and inform everyone, at every level of the facility/organization, of the changes associated with CPOE implementation. This champion must coordinate with all other champion groups to ensure continuity and consistency throughout the lifecycle of the project. The process starts with the champion assessing current communication tools and their effectiveness with each of the stakeholder groups. In addition, this champion pays particular attention on the right communication based on the level of impact on each stakeholder group.

One may define communication as high, low, or medium impact. High impact implies significant change in the end-user's workflow or thought processes. Low impact implies that the associated change is minimal. Medium impact implies it is neither high nor low. As the team develops messages, either before or even after CPOE activation, the Communication Champion determines which level of impact that message will be to each stakeholder group.

For example, the team's invitation to attend the CPOE kick-off event is a low impact communication and requires only a low impact communication technique, such as a flyer or announcement on the unit. However, if one stakeholder group tends to skip events like this, we would categorize their communication as medium and follow the flyer with a personal invitation (or stronger encouragement) coming from the manager or director over that area. The kick-off event itself, however, represents a high impact opportunity, as it will create major workflow changes and new job descriptions. Therefore, one should make this a "town-hall" type of event and ask the CEO to lead it. At this event, the CEO will elicit questions and have direct dialogue with the participants. Employees and physician who attend will have questions, and the town hall is an excellent format for dialogue. The author also recommends that the CEO host multiple kick-off events, including at least one in the evening for the night shift employees. Moreover, during these events, the change manager will take notes on all questions. The team will later post these questions and their answers on the FAQ (Frequently Asked Questions) on the CPOE Knowledge Repository.

During the CRA, the Communication Champion takes the lead in helping the facility's CPOE team in creating a theme for their CPOE project. The theme should be fun and relate to the facility and its CPOE goals. Once the group selects the theme, the Communication Champion works on developing the messages, flyers and templates and presents the ideas to the other champions. If all agree, then everyone leverages the facility's theme in every event, every communication, as well as all project paraphernalia, such as lanyards and T-shirts. Commonly, the Director of Marketing assumes the role of Communications Champion.

Collaborating with the Stakeholder Champion above, the Communication Champion owns the materials, tools and resources to articulate the "What's in it for me?" message at each event and to each stakeholder group. Together, these two champions ensure that they identify, inform and engage all CPOE-impacted audiences (stakeholder groups). They work to minimize confusion, surprises, resistance and misinformation, which helps these groups to obtain buy-in for CPOE. The Communication Champion finds and documents answers to the following key questions:

- How does the facility current communicate to the various stakeholders, such as staff, patients and physicians?
- What communication vehicles does the facility already use? What is the target audience of each? Are the current communication vehicles effective with the stakeholders?
- What are the key messages that the team will communicate during the project?
- Who should communicate these messages? When should the team deliver the messages?
- How will stakeholders provide feedback during this project?
- How will we make the FAQs available?

To achieve a successful engagement, the champion will write a Communication Plan that includes timelines, communication vehicles, owners, and target audiences for each. You usually want them to include articles in their employee newsletter, flyers, "elevator speeches." committee updates, town halls, as well as external communications to patients and media. The champion creates content for all communications, which she directs to what will be happening in the next 30 days. The champion designs low impact (non-interactive) messages that she delivers using one-way communication vehicles such as e-mail, flyers, newsletters or web site postings. However, even low impact messages should allow the user an avenue for questions such as a contact person, e-mail address, or link to the FAQ site. The communication team creates medium and high impact messaging opportunities that permit the end-users to have interactive dialogue and real-time feedback.

The "elevator speech", with a monthly theme, exemplifies the medium impact communication tool. The Communication Champion each month distributes a 30–60 s message to the executives and champions that promotes the CPOE activities/goals of the next 30 days. They actively look for opportunities to deliver this message, when in the elevator, cafeteria, or briefly at the informal times before or after meetings. These create opportunities for short dialogues and demonstrate to stakeholders that everyone is on the same page. In addition, committee chairpersons should also see every meeting as an opportunity to update their members on the CPOE project and the impact to their area of responsibility.

The pulse survey is another important tool this team uses to measure the effectiveness of the communication plan. We recommend that the Communication Champion distribute a survey about every 6 weeks. We used the following questions during the AHS engagements:

Pulse Survey (1–5: scored – Strongly Disagree, Disagree, Neutral, Agree, or Strongly Agree)

- Staff and physicians are aware that change is coming with Computerized Physician Order Entry (CPOE).
- Staff and physicians understand why we are making this change.
- Our communications about this project have been effective.
- Leadership is appropriately addressing the needs of the organization as related to the CPOE project.
- The general feeling of the facility related to this project is positive.

Two free-text questions:

- What questions are people asking about this project?
- What would you do if you were the person responsible for the success of this project?

The pulse survey is anonymous and provides an average score for each designated stakeholder group. We bar graph the score for each survey and present the results regularly at the monthly Champion meetings. The team uses the two free-text responses to update the FAQ, to select content for upcoming communications and town halls, and adjust the Stakeholder Engagement Plan as needed. A team goal should be the improvement in the average scores for each question, each time they administer the pulse survey.

There are many signs of not having an effective Communication Plan. Rumor, hearsay and innuendo permeate the project environment, leading to chaos.

Stakeholder groups may create unnecessary resistance and the majority of end-users remain disconnected from the project. The effective communication process ensures that project leaders are successfully communicating with all end-users, from staff, physicians, and the community, and that they are building their facility's excitement and buy-in throughout the process.

5.16 Training

The Training Champion should be the executive (other than the CEO) who has the best record of accomplishment for holding accountability throughout all levels of the organization. This champion is responsible to oversee the training plan, and meet all training goals prior to CPOE activation. The champion typically has an operational structure around training, in the form of a training department, a training manager, or a team of educators. For CPOE, however, the facility has to grow the infrastructure and effectively staff enough trainers and proctors for every employee and provider to complete all aspects of training, competency, and practice.

The goal of the Training Champion is to ensure that all end-users, including all providers, have appropriately trained to perform their responsibilities within a CPOE environment. Success does not end at completion of training, but that the end-users are fully leveraging CPOE to reduce patient harm, with improved efficiency and maximal effectiveness (i.e. improved outcomes and less waste and duplication). The author discusses physician training in more detail in a later chapter.

This champion focuses on forming the team to author and execute a training plan, while he maintains accountability over all aspects of the plan. This champion needs to stay out of the weeds while holding everyone accountable to the plan. To maintain credibility, this champion completes his own training as early as possible, not only to make a statement, but also to ensure the program maintains effectiveness and quality. Moreover, the champion expects all members of the management team to be the first to train within their departments. This ensures that each member of the management team is leading by example, as well as fully prepared to understand the future state of CPOE workflows within their areas of responsibility.

Within a formal Training Plan, the champion approves the outline of all course materials, class format and the time schedules for each stakeholder/departmental group who will train for CPOE. This includes training of all providers. The training team will also track training statistics, separating out employees by department and providers. We typically recommend that the facility work with the Medical Staff Office coordinator to stratify physicians by level of activity within the hospital. While all providers must complete training prior to seeing any patient once CPOE is live, one should especially want to track the physicians who regularly attend to patients in the hospital. AHS defined "tier 1" physicians as those who have five or more encounters (admissions, consultations or operations) in a typical month, and "tier 2" physicians as those who have less. The author recommends that you track employees by department and physicians by these tiers, or similar designations. Many will also want to track employed/contracted physicians within their areas of responsibility, such as Emergency Physicians, Hospitalists or Radiologists, while others track by specialty (Cardiology, General Surgery, and Anesthesiology). At academic centers, we track residents, medical students, fellows and attending physician staff separately.

As mentioned above, the Training Champion will work with the change manager to create the Learning Plan during the CRA phase of the project.

The Training Champion should determine the answers to the following key questions:

- What will be the format for training for each stakeholder group or role?
- What will be the length of training for each role?
- Where will training occur?
- What materials and tools will you use for training?
- How will we determine competencies?
- How much time will we allocate to end-users practicing?

The champion will incorporate answers to each of the above into the formal Training Plan. This plan includes course outlines, specific curricula, training aids, and plans for determining competencies. The champion will collaborate with the Workflow Champion to ensure that training incorporates all information that the latter has approved in his Start/Stop/Continue Document. At least 1 month prior to training begins, the champion will approve the training schedule for each role and distribute that to all members of the management team.

The Training Champion also ensures that someone is accountable to communicate training schedules for the providers and track their progress. Typically, the coordinator of the Medical Staff Office already has effective processes for communication to all members of the Medical Staff. However, it usually takes a village to communicate training requirements, schedule class times and follow up with no shows with the providers. One typically sees the Chief Medical Officer (or other named physician on the executive team), Medical Staff Office, trainers and physician informatics support team working together to complete the training of these critical end-users.

The risks of not having an effective training plan include a poor implementation with end-users demonstrating confusion and resistance. While some projects fail completely when the team executes poorly, the effort to turn around the others is enormous. Organizations should have a great training plan to leverage the full benefits of CPOE.

5.17 Workflow

The Workflow Champion leads one of the larger teams with the goal to optimize CPOE processes so that each department and stakeholder group achieves clinical, financial and operational excellence. This Champion aligns with our third principle of informatics, "Automating broken processes get us to the wrong place faster." Like the Training Champion, this champion probably needs to be a vice president or senior director due to the level of accountability that this person needs to maintain throughout the project. CPOE and the resultant seamless flow of orders and information, breaks down many silos within the facility and forces departments to consider how their processes affect the other departments. It takes a strong workflow champion to overcome the inertia of these silos. Therefore, this champion must have strong influence and authority within the organization to be successful.

In a single hospital implementation, most of the workflow design occurs in the early phases of the project when it is critical for proper system design (see Chap. 4). In the multi-hospital system, the Workflow Champion must work within the system design and translate that to the end-user processes. Regardless of when workflow design occurs, the champion should ensure that actual end-users contribute to workflow documentation and design. Successes comes when one considers what end-users actually do in their daily roles rather than what management believes they do. The Workflow Champion oversees and reports workflow progress at the monthly Champion meetings. The champion will have multiple leaders to lead workflow redesign efforts for the numerous processes of CPOE. The typical structure is for the champion to create a Workflow Redesign Team with multiple working groups below them to address specific objectives and processes. We have touched on these major processes in Chap. 4.

The Workflow Champion obtains and documents the answers to the following key questions:

• What key processes does CPOE affect?
• What is the gap between current (what we do now) and future (what we will do) states for each process?
• Which paper-based processes will we automate during our CPOE project?
• Which processes will we not automate?
• To what extent do we affect stakeholder groups and roles with CPOE?
• Which workflows will we specifically target for improvement/enhancement rather than wait for post-implementation (i.e. optimization) efforts?
• How will the end-users best leverage CPOE content and evidence-based practice?

Regardless of when the team addresses workflow design, the Workflow Champion is responsible for several activities and deliverables:

• List of key processes impacted by CPOE, including current and future-state process maps.
• Create a list of key processes that will remain on paper after you implement CPOE.
• Any pre-implementation workflows that you will introduce, such as new evidence-based order sets, to help end-users familiarize themselves with content. Often you can introduce these new order sets on paper to encourage the providers to become early adopters.

- Communicate any pre-implementation policies/practices that you will introduce prior to implementation to correct current broken processes.
- Create a list of rules/alerts that you will implement to address specific patient safety or regulatory goals.
- The Workflow Champion ensures that each department, role and/or stakeholder group contributes to the Start/Stop/Continue Document (SSC Document).
- Collaborates with the Training Champion to ensure end-users complete training with competency, not only around system functionality, but also around the appropriate CPOE workflows with full understanding of the SSC Document.

Ultimately, the Workflow Champion ensures their team identifies and addresses all workflow processes that will change with CPOE. When the organization under-emphasizes workflow redesign, it tends to achieve less efficient and effective processes, and end up with the consequences of automating their broken processes. As a result, poorly executed CPOE will frustrate you employees and your medical staff, and fail to achieve the outcomes that you desire. It is critical that the leadership understand and commit to every aspect of the change management program for a successful CPOE project.

5.18 Performance Management

The Performance Management Champion bears the responsibility to confirm that CPOE brings measureable results to the organization. The ideal champion has a passion for data and outcomes. One should typically encourage a vice president (i.e. executive leader) in this role. The author has seen Chief Financial Officers (CFO), Chief Nursing Officers (CNO) and Chief Medical or Quality Officers (CMO or CQO) become successful Performance Management Champions. For large health systems, one typically looks at both facility outcomes as well as health system outcomes. In this scenario, the local champion will focus on local outcomes only and use the health system data as a benchmark.

Since CPOE creates an opportunity to implement new processes/workflows, skills, attitudes and behaviors, this champion wants to determine objectively that they have eliminated errors, waste and unnecessary variance. In addition, CPOE should increase the adoption of evidence-based content, provide effective clinical decision support, reduce medication errors and thereby reduce the risk of patient harm. The author also recommends that the Performance Management Champion continue regular reporting of CPOE outcomes to the Board, the Medical Staff, the employees and the patients.

Over the years, the author has seen much variation in what organizations and single hospitals want to measure as part of the CPOE project. In order to facilitate the discussion, he has divided the opportunities into two categories, metrics (process measures) and analytics (outcome measures). He defines metrics as those measurements that occur because of end-users simply using the CPOE system. Some examples of these metrics include:

- Number and percent of all orders entered by CPOE providers
- Number and percent of medication orders entered by CPOE providers
- Number of clinical decision support (CDS) alerts that fire to a provider
- The percent of CDS alerts that change provider ordering[8] as compared to overridden
- The usage (number and possibly percentage use) of evidence-based order sets
- The number of documents which providers create electronically
- Error trapping, such as detecting inaccuracy of order entry such as nurses entering verbal/phone orders as written/CPOE orders into the EMR[9]

The author defines analytics as comparative measurements within the organization that determine whether a new process has allowed the end-user to produce a measureable improvement in an outcome. Unlike the metrics above, the Performance Management Team needs to collect baseline measurements prior to CPOE in order to create a post-CPOE outcome. Some specific examples of these analytics include:

- Improvement in turn-around time of stat laboratory tests and common imaging studies
- Reduction in adverse drug events (ADEs) as well as reduction in ADE which cause harm/death
- Reduction in overall cost per case
- Reduction in pharmacy/laboratory cost per case
- Reduction in all-cause mortality
- Improvement in quality measures scores
- Reduction in surgical infections
- Decrease in time to complete admission processes
- Decrease in time to complete discharge processes
- Improvement in medication reconciliation rates
- Improvement in specific employee/departmental processes such as time nurses spend charting, physician rounding, or inter-unit transfers

The major challenge in measuring analytic data is the work one must do to collect the baseline data prior to CPOE. In many cases, the pre-CPOE processes are paper-based, and require considerable cost for the organization to abstract

---

[8] When it comes to many alerts, providers can accept the alert and cancel the order, modify the order (e.g. change a dose or frequency of a medication), order an additional intervention (e.g. order a lab test as a follow up as recommended by the alert), or override the alert and document a reason that the alert does not apply to this patient, for example.

[9] The consequence of this scenario is the EMR should electronically route verbal/phone orders to a provider for co-signature. If the nurse taking the order enters it inappropriately, it may not route for co-signing and become an order that a physician has not authenticated. This behavior needs immediate reeducation and accountability, as there are often regulatory or financial implications when physicians fail to sign/authenticate orders in a timely fashion.

the baseline data. Therefore, many organizations forego a lengthy pre-CPOE assessment and pick one or two analytic measures to address prior to implementation.

Taking the time to measure your CPOE metrics and analytics, however creates an opportunity to affirm your successful efforts and to modify areas where you are not achieving the intended results. In addition, purposely measuring your processes helps you to create awareness of what you hope to achieve.

The Performance Management Champion should address the following key questions:

- What determines our project team's success?
- From the leadership point of view, what determines CPOE success and how do we measure it?
- From the staff and physician points of view, what determines CPOE success and how do we measure it?
- How do we measure employee performance on processes we plan to target for improvement?
- How do we plan to tie performance of the individual to the performance of the unit, department or hospital?
- What are the best returns on investment (ROI) opportunities for our CPOE project?
- Where do employees need to perform new processes/workflows, exhibit new behaviors, or develop new skill sets?
- How will we incentivize new processes, skills and behaviors?

The Performance Management Champion should have defined activities and deliverables for the selected CPOE metrics and analytics and collaborate with the Director of Human Resources and Employee Impact Champion on suggesting opportunities for employee incentives. The champion will want to ascertain key performance indicators such as employee productivity, measured against baseline and/or health system, regional or industry benchmarks. The two may also choose to collaborate on new employee performance evaluations, which are more pertinent to new CPOE roles and workflow.

It is also important that the champion share both metric and analytic data on a timely fashion. The author agrees with the old adage that "What gets measured, get better!" For example, ordering errors start occurring as you implement CPOE. It is crucial that this champion provides timely error data to management, so that they may correct employee errors and reinforce best practices. Early intervention to training and knowledge gaps helps employees and physicians to learn the correct processes and steps before the errors become otherwise habitual.

It is a fine balance between how much process improvement and measurement one does prior CPOE and the opportunities to refine data after CPOE is live. While most pre-CPOE data is paper-based, the CPOE environment is very data rich and affords the Performance Management Champion endless opportunities for measurement and optimization of processes and workflow.

5.19 Employee Impact

The Employee Impact Champion focuses on the human resources aspects of change throughout the CPOE project, especially the retention of key employees in the process. The Director of Human Resources typically serves in this role. This champion is a key collaborator with other champions as they collectively plan engagement strategies, communication and changes in workflow. As a result, the Employee Impact Champion is committed to eliminate unnecessary processes and provide opportunities for employees to learn new skills. This champion also works with the management team to rewrite job descriptions in addition to retaining top talent in the organization.

Without this focus, employees (e.g. hospital unit clerks or HUCs) fear job elimination, obsolescence and productivity loss. Instead, this champion should help the team identify and promote the "What's in it for me?" message to high-risk employees. This may include specific incentives for key employees associated with project success. Therefore, this champion should understand the job impact to various roles during the planning and implementation of CPOE. In addition, the champion must understand the skills, knowledge and competencies that employees may need in the CPOE environment. Finally, the champion should develop a strategy to retain key employees. Retention strategies may include communication, compensation/incentives and career development. The champion addresses the following key questions around employee impact:

- Who are the critical CPOE team members?
- How will the hospital retain key project members?
- Which employees will have significant change to their workflow and competencies because of workflow redesign around CPOE?
- What is the affect to recruitment, orientation, training, and ongoing assessment of employees in the high-risk roles?

The Employee Impact Champion will identify the key, non-executive members of the CPOE project team and assess their individual needs for training, recognition and advancement. Then he will collaborate with the management team on updating job descriptions and evaluations for those, such as HUCs, whose will experience major role changes. This champion will also regularly review the stakeholder analysis and engagement plans as well as the efforts of the workflow redesign teams. The goal is to bring employees along through the CPOE process and leave no one behind.

5.20 Knowledge Management

The Knowledge Management Champion organizes and manages the tools, calendars, information and knowledge for the CPOE project. For single hospital projects, this individual also manages the CPOE order sets, clinical decision support documentation and posting of CPOE policies. This champion determines a defined process for collecting, indexing and archiving the tools and work product of the project. In most cases, she will collaborate with the local owner of the facility's intranet website for this purpose. Many facilities already have a website content owner who may become the best choice for the champion role.

The goal of this champion is allow management and end-users to quickly access information about the project, including all presentations, non-confidential tools, workflow diagrams, survey results, FAQs and calendar of events. The site should not risk this information residing only on the hard drive of one computer. Moreover, the champion should align the information repository with the theme of project. Many teams also include a countdown clock to designate the time left until CPOE activation.

The Knowledge Management Champion should assess the project needs and create a defined process for knowledge capture, archiving and sharing. The champion should have the site live before the end of the CRA phase so that it can be fully functional and useful by the CPOE Kick-Off event. Once the web team establishes the site during the CRA phase, this champion should need less than 1 h/week to maintain.

At AHS, the CPOE team also established a corporate CPOE site with information useful to all our hospitals. We discuss this in further detail in Chap. 6.

5.21 Executive and Leadership Coaching

The author has evolved this position over the years to represent more than a traditional hospital executive sponsor. The ideal person for this role is the CEO. In academic medical centers and large community hospitals, however, the COO may actually run the hospital day-to-day. The author has worked with several projects through the years with the COO in this role. This champion keeps the management team engaged and focused on the project and the associated change. In addition, the Coaching Champion may see opportunities for members of the management team to improve their skills around major change initiatives. This champion is the go-to person for the change manager when the wheels are falling off the project bus.

This champion should consider the following key questions:

- Do any members of the leadership team require new behaviors or skills to lead change?
- Do end-users and middle management trust the leadership team's ability to lead change?
- What are the best resources and opportunities to support the project champions in their roles?

The champion should work with the change manager to understand the role of the other champions, and monitor and assist any that fall behind or are not accountable to their project responsibilities. This champion often does ongoing education and training during biweekly or monthly leadership meetings. He is continually assessing the leadership's capacity and commitment toward successful CPOE. As he identifies gaps in any leader's skills or participation, he develops strategies to address them immediately.

The Executive and Leadership Coaching champion encourages improved skill sets of the leadership in the area of managing change. This provides confidence in the management's team ability to manage all the change of CPOE. The leaders become visibly involved and take ownership of the CPOE change process. Ultimately, the leaders exhibit high accountability for CPOE and grow in their change management knowledge for future projects/initiatives.

5.22 Patient/Community Engagement

The executive team selects the Patient/Community Champion to represent the interests of the patient throughout the CPOE process. This is a particularly important role in the single hospital project. The champion should be a person who neither works for the hospital nor is the spouse of an employee or physician. Often the executives select a Board Member who can commit to the project and has no other healthcare background. Ideally, the champion attends the initial CRA Executive Workshop to get an introduction to CPOE, and thereafter attends the Kick-off event and the monthly Champion meetings. The main purpose of this role is to represent the interests of the patient in all discussions. The CEO should ask this champion to write a few paragraphs for the employee newsletter about her impression of the CPOE project. In addition, the champion may have opportunities to promote the hospital and its CPOE initiative at community events.

5.23 Physician Engagement

Since physicians are key stakeholders for CPOE, it is important that the facility have several physicians engaged in the project. They typically participate in order set content development and review, clinical decision support development and occasionally shepherd provider training. There also may be a physician on the executive team, as Chief Medical Officer, Vice President of Medical Affairs, or as a service line director. The author has listed the characteristics one should look for in a physician champion:

5.23.1 Physician Champion Characteristics

- Respected for leadership and communication skills and clinical role modeling
- Actively involved in direct inpatient care & having excellent practice outcomes

- Passionate/enthusiastic to achieve high quality performance indicators and process improvements
- Willing to devote time, energy and activism to make changes
- Seeks to understand current processes, data and outcomes
- Brings personal vision and innovation to the table
- Troubleshooter; and resource for problem-solving

5.23.2   Physician Champion Skills

- Masters CPOE & electronic documentation skills, serving as coach and communicator to medical staff and departmental peers through completion of computer-based training and instruction
- Is an advanced user of the EMR prior to CPOE activation

5.23.3   Physician Champion Responsibilities

- Serve on local Physician Informatics Committee
- Adjust schedule to attend monthly CPOE Champion meetings and represents medical staff interests
- Participate actively on team, project meetings and project exercises
- Trains and guides the Super-users on the patient floors before and after the conversion
- Advocates CPOE among peers and during medical staff meetings
- Familiarizes self with CPOE literature and business case including national initiatives for adoption

The executive team should contract in writing with the Physician Champion(s) prior to any work on the project and ideally, prior to the Executive CRA Workshop. The executive team and physician determine if there will be any honorarium for participation. If so, the author recommends it be on an hourly basis with a plan to track and formally submit time and expenses to the CFO.

5.23.4   CMO/Medical Director

- Helps facilitate MEC (Medical Executive Committee) in forming a Physician Informatics Committee if it does not already exist. Serves as *ex officio* member of physician informatics committee and provides broad-based input for transformation of the hospital to CPOE.

- Engages patient care providers with varying roles including physicians, nursing practitioners, nursing staff, ancillary department personnel, and medical records professionals to contribute to the development and use of the clinical information systems
- Develops empathy and understanding of physician needs and builds relationships with physicians to gain support of IT initiatives and the migration of hospital to CPOE and online documentation
- Reviews medical informatics trends, experiences and approaches, develops technical and application implementation strategies and assists in the development of strategic plans at both hospital and corporate level for clinical information systems projects
- Collaborates with the CMIO and other clinical leaders to implement CPOE and related clinical systems
- Establishes and maintains an ongoing discussion to orient and develop provider buy-in for CPOE with Chiefs of Staff, members of the Medical Executive Committee, Clinical Chiefs, and other medical staff leaders in the hospital
- Engages and works in concert with Physician champions to assure wide spread acceptance and provider use of the CPOE and other electronic clinical systems
- Actively participates in physician CPOE training classes and competencies
- Actively supports the CPOE activation for first 90 days

The author discusses specific physician engagement strategy and techniques in Chap. 7.

5.24 Key Points

- Change management addresses the people aspect of the CPOE project
- An organization needs a defined change management plan for CPOE
- The change management plan begins with a CPOE Readiness Assessment
- Key areas of change management for the CPOE project include stakeholder engagement, communication, training, workflow redesign, employee impact, knowledge management, leadership coaching in addition to physician engagement
- The organization should designate key leaders to serve as champions during the CPOE project
- Each area of change management have defined benefits as well as risks if the leadership does not address

5.25 Fingernails on the Chalkboard

- **"Oh, the project manager also does change management."**
  Every clinical project that involves IT and transformation of care will need to address people, process, and technology. The project manager owns scope,

timelines and resource management of the endeavor. The change manager focuses on the people and workflow aspects of the project. Due to the complexity of CPOE, it takes both competent project and change management for success. Often one person cannot facilitate all the activities nor have all the necessary skills and tools for success.

- **"Oh, change management; our training department does that."**
While training is an important piece of the change management pie, the overall change management effort begins in the executive suite and includes important responsibilities in addition to training. Typically, the training resources are not equipped to perform a CPOE readiness assessment, manage workflow redesign or create a communication plan. An organization that focuses only on training will miss the many benefits of a comprehensive change management strategy and plan.

- **"Change management is the fluff of the project."**
This is a common statement at the start of a CPOE, often coming from both the executive suites and the IT team. However, once these individuals experience a CPOE implementation with effective change management, they typically change their minds and want to incorporate a change management plan into future projects.

- **"CPOE is not very intuitive"**
This is a true statement, which end-users, and especially physicians, often repeat as they start to experience CPOE. They use it as a rationale to complain as they resist the change from hand-written orders. The facts are that healthcare and direct patient care represent a complex business, and not as simple as downloading a new application onto the latest tablet device. Just as we would never let a surgeon perform an operation without training and practice, we should never implement CPOE without directed efforts at end-user engagement, workflow redesign, extensive training, practice, and assurance of competency. The goal is not to intuitively move end-users from paper charts and processes to their electronic versions. The goal is to transform patient care. All end-users, including the physicians, need specific preparation and training for CPOE to safe, efficient and effective.

- **The organization begins to see increasing signs and symptoms of active or passive resistance among key stakeholders**
All CPOE projects will experience end-users exhibiting both active and passive resistance early in the project. However, your communication plan and stakeholder engagement should actively build the case for CPOE and help them to find the "What's in it for me?" answers. If end-user resistance is growing, the champions need to reassess their plan. Common problems include:

1. Lack of visibility of the senior executives
2. Too much one-way communication and not enough two-way dialogue
3. Inconsistent leadership messaging
4. Too many competing projects/priorities
5. Ineffective CPOE Champions

The hospital CPOE champions should meet with executive leaders and review their activities against their written action plans. The executive sponsor should evaluate whether the right individuals are in the right roles for the project. The team makes course adjustments as needed to reenergize and refocus the project.

Chapter 6
CPOE Change Readiness Assessment

Abstract This chapter takes the concept of the Change Readiness Assessment which the author introduced in the previous chapter and lays out the specific content of each step of the first 90 days of a CPOE engagement. The chapter also includes the specific content of the executive workshop. The author also presents how their team assesses the organizational culture and the tools they use in that process.

> *If you always do what you've always done, you'll always get what you've always got*
>
> *– Anonymous*

Since 2001, the author has experienced much value through performing a formal CPOE Readiness Assessment (CRA) during the 90 days before facility kick-off of a CPOE project. This phase begins with an initial workshop, specific stakeholder interviews, a formal survey of organizational culture and various change management activities to lead up to the facility kick-off event. These latter activities include the project leadership reviewing the CRA with the management team; a communication assessment; a facility learning assessment; initial stakeholder analysis; and employee retention assessment. Every aspect of the first 90 days allows the CPOE leadership team to assess the climate and culture of the facility. The CPOE Steering Committee and the facility leadership leverage the CPOE Readiness Assessment to identify specific, local project risks and determine an appropriate CPOE activation date. Since the author has seen much value and effectiveness in the Executive CRA Workshop, he will describe the actual components of the CRA in detail below.

P.A. Smith, *Making Computerized Provider Order Entry Work*,
Health Information Technology Standards,
DOI 10.1007/978-1-4471-4243-0_6, © Springer-Verlag London 2013

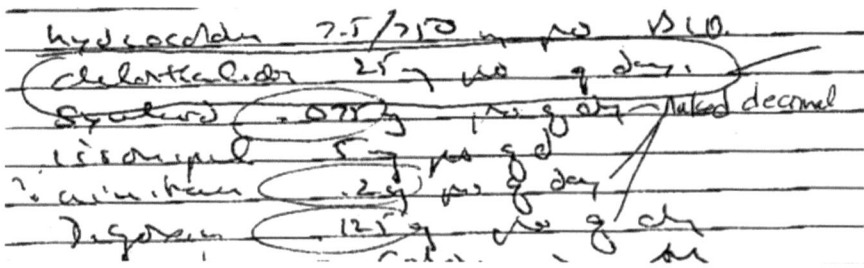

Fig. 6.1 Example of typical handwritten inpatient orders. *Circles* indicate decimals with no leading zero

6.1   The Executive CRA Workshop

The CPOE leadership team[1] presents the Executive CRA Workshop at the facility with the entire facility executive team[2] in attendance. In addition, the facility invites most directors[3] as well as personnel with key responsibilities for CPOE. It is important that it is an interactive event, so one arranges the tables in a U formation, open at the projector screen end. The CPOE team often arrives to find the room arranged classroom or auditorium style, and will quickly rearrange the seating to encourage collaboration. Each member of the CPOE team sits at different vantage points in the room to observe body language and assess the attendees dynamics of participation in the event. The workshop lasts a full 4 h.

After introductions, the CPOE team begins their event with an icebreaker exercise. Your exercise should be consistent with your organizational culture and not create any barriers to participation. At AHS, Charol Martindale, our clinical applications director, devised an icebreaker in which she gives each facility participant an index card and asks each to write down "two things you hope CPOE achieves at this facility and one thing you hope it doesn't." She then collects the cards, then reads them off, asking the group to identify whom they believe the author is. We tally the comments and achieve several helpful outcomes from the exercise: We hear what each person's hopes and fears are for CPOE, and we get to observe how well they know one another and interact. The participants seem to have fun with this exercise, and it really helps to have those hopes and fears on the table at the start. Previously, the author has utilized various other ice-breakers. However, the icebreaker should be appropriate to the audience.

---

[1] Typically, this team includes the Executive Sponsor, the Medical Director, Clinical Applications Director, IT Director, Informatics Lead and the Change Manager.

[2] The team schedules the event so that every member of the C-Suite (CEO, COO, CFO, CNO and CMO) attends. We recommend you not hold the event otherwise.

[3] Typically, the directors include human resources, critical care, nursing, pharmacy, emergency department, surgery, patient financial services, information technology, and health information management. Other attendees include any physician champions, the community champion and the local informatics support including those who directly support the physicians.

Next, the workshop introduces an overview of CPOE and workflows. The author actually makes the point to define CPOE as "the providers actually putting orders directly into the EMR and the addition of clinical decision support during the ordering process." On should repeatedly stress the patient safety aspects of CPOE, especially the reduction in medication errors and administration delays.

Then you should introduce our anchor slide, as demonstrated in Fig. 6.1, first showing the current state of written orders as below:

This example allows us to discuss some key issues with handwritten orders:

- Illegibility, leading not only to guesses by nurses and pharmacists, but delays in the patient receiving the initial dose of the medication. One may choose to embellish it with the image of a group of nurses standing around trying to figure out what Dr. Smith really ordered until one has a brilliant idea, "Let's fax it up to the pharmacist and let him figure it out!"
- Wrong dose, especially as we point out that the fifth medication is in grams, while the sixth medication is in milligrams, though they look identical.
- Regulatory issues, as in the case of the leading zeros.
- Callbacks, in that eventually the nurse may have to call the doctor back and obtain clarity on the order. Moreover, the doctor may now be in the office and no longer has the immediate context of the patient on which the nurse is questioning the order. Meanwhile, the patient is not receiving the medication ordered.

From there we introduce the future state by showing the CPOE version of the orders immediately underneath the handwritten orders as in Fig. 6.2:

Even laypersons can clearly see the difference between handwritten orders and electronic orders. In the first case, the pharmacist or nurse determines the physician's intent in the handwritten order. In the EMR example, the physician clearly orders the intended drug with the specific dose, route and frequency as well as the benefits from immediate clinical alerts if appropriate.

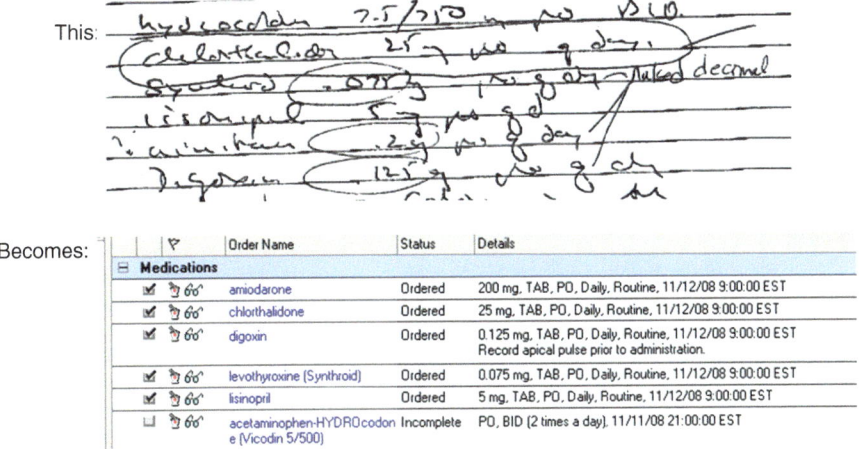

Fig. 6.2 CPOE order in place of handwritten version

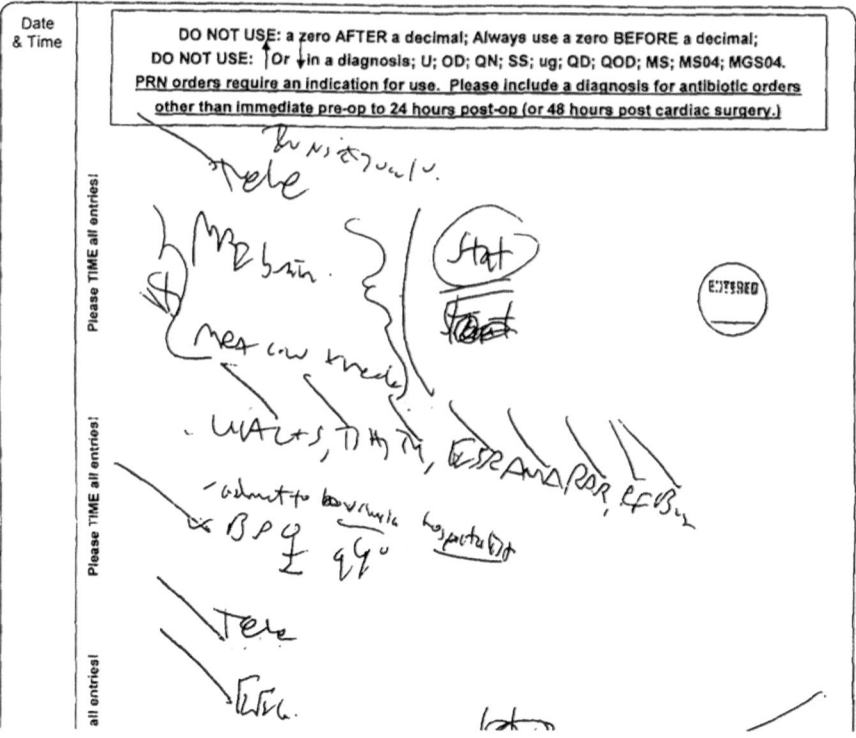

Fig. 6.3 Example of handwritten Stat orders. Note the lack of time stamp despite multiple reminders on the page

There is a hidden message in the example that only one person pointed out in 3 years that the author used this particular example. The first handwritten order is either hydrocodone 7.5/750 mg (probably intended as acetaminophen dose of 750 mg with 7.5 mg hydrocodone) or hydrocodone cough syrup. The person interpreting the order has represented it as Vicodin 5/500 (5 mg hydrocodone with 500 mg acetaminophen) with a missing dose instruction of 1.5 tablets twice a day. So in fact, the author had purposely created a transcription error to represent how such errors happen every day in the world of handwritten orders.

However, it was only a matter of time until one of our sites submitted the Stat orders below (Fig. 6.3) that a physician ironically wrote 2 days prior to CPOE go live at his facility.

As the author discussed in an earlier chapter, he uses these images of orders to state a strong case for the electronic order as "source of truth." This represents the concept of an anchor for the vision of patient safety. One does not have to be a healthcare veteran to understand the clarity, accuracy and efficiency that occurs when the physician writes his order electronically, rather than having someone transcribe the handwritten orders.

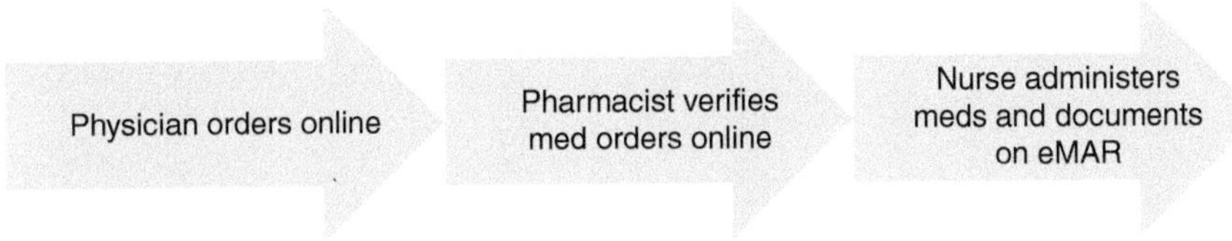

Fig. 6.4 CPOE Process (The Obvious). This demonstrates how many initially visualize the impact of CPOE, as only affecting the physicians, the pharmacists and the nurses around the medication process

After introducing our anchor images, the presenter shows a flow chart with swim lanes (i.e. showing process steps broken down by roles) to demonstrate the complexity of the medication order processes with handwritten orders as compared to the CPOE future state. The future state shows the addition of CDS, the elimination of the HUC in the process, and a reduction in time between the physician's medication order and the administration time. Again, they stay on task of reinforcing patient safety, efficiency and effectiveness.

The team then discusses their project goals for CPOE. At AHS, they set the bar that physicians would enter more than 80 % of the medication orders (i.e. less than 20 % verbal/telephone orders), leverage evidence-based order set content, produce a large amount of documentation online using structured concepts, and benefit from an integrated discharge process that would produce patient discharge instructions as a byproduct of the physician's discharge documentation. Many organizations set various other goals for CPOE.

The presenter then moves to the discussion to CPOE workflow. It really starts by showing a simple diagram (Fig. 6.4) that represents how most people envision CPOE initially. The author likes to call this, "CPOE Processes (The Obvious)."

Many healthcare leaders and employees initially have a limited understanding of how CPOE will affect their workflow. In fact, the author hears repeatedly that their biggest concern is how the doctors will accept putting orders into the computer. However, when one really understands all the processes downstream to each order, the process diagram becomes more complex. We like to call the subsequent diagram (Fig. 6.5), "CPOE Processes (The Reality)."

The author typically presents many actual CPOE stories to illustrate some of these CPOE processes. He has used similar diagrams for other CPOE projects. He finds that it helps both the leaders and end-users understand that "CPOE affects almost every process in the hospital. Therefore, CPOE affects everything and everyone in the hospital. And, as we know, everyone resists change; resulting in stress, change in behaviors, acting out and complaining." He then concludes this discussion with reviewing a few specific changes that physicians experience in their workflows, such as ordering, documentation, admission/discharge/transfer processes, and complying with regulatory standards.

After completing the workflow discussions, the team presents any online repository of CPOE resources. A single facility should create and manage an online site of all

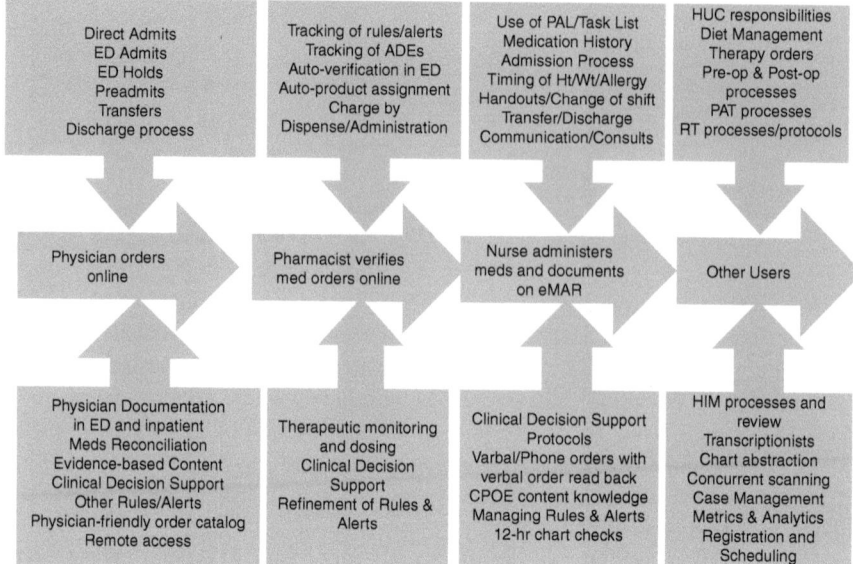

Fig. 6.5 CPOE Processes (The Reality). This demonstrates a few of the multidisciplinary processes that CPOE affects

materials, references and schedules. Since AHS had multiple CPOE activations to manage, it became practical to create a single intranet site to host the team resources for the sites. The AHS CPOE team called their site *CPOE 511*, a kind of "one stop shopping" site on their corporate intranet, with hyperlinks to it from the intranet home pages of every hospital. While the content of each document is specific to the facility or organization, the structure may be helpful to sites wishing to create one of their own.

- **FAQs** (Frequently asked questions). As one pilots CPOE, one should keep records of every question that employees and physicians ask, and compile them with your answers. New team members also find benefits from this searchable list of common questions and their answers.
- **Press Kit**. Since every hospital wants to promote their activation of CPOE, your communication team should consider a press kit with general information on CPOE, the health system, and pertinent quotes and outcomes on the project. In addition, at AHS, the communication team interviewed physicians from their first five CPOE sites and produced a compelling video of CPOE testimonials to show to their future CPOE sites.
- **Workflow diagrams**. During the rollout of CPOE, it is important that you maintain a library of various current state (i.e. Pre-CPOE) workflow as well as your future state workflows. We used Microsoft Visio and their basic flow sheets with swim lanes by role to consistently document and communicate our current and future state workflows. Once a team completes a pair of workflow diagrams, they produce a Start/Stop/Continue document by department to clearly state, "What

you will start doing when CPOE goes live?" "What will you stop doing once CPOE goes live?" and "What will you continue to do?" once CPOE is live. You should also provide information on downtime processes.

- **CPOE Policies**. At AHS, we manage hyperlinks from CPOE 511, directly to our CPOE policies, similar to those the author discussed in an earlier chapter.
- **Order Set Repository**. One should keep a complete, up-to-date list of all standardized and local order sets as well as an order set repository, which physicians can access during system downtimes.
- **Clinical Reference Library**. This refers to your online library of pertinent CPOE articles, such as the ones you reference during presentations as well as those the various CPOE content committees utilize for their order sets. You may also provide links from your order sets, directly into evidence-based references such as Zynx Health.
- **Presentations**. Whether you are a single facility or a health system, it is beneficial to post all your standard presentations on the intranet. This library of presentations not only includes presentations giving during the formal project events, but also brief promotions to use during departmental meetings and other occasions.
- **Tip and Tricks**. Over time you will develop numerous tips and tricks to help end-users become more efficient, to solve specific issues or to introduce new features or functionality. At AHS, they also include information on using touch-pad devices and smart phones to access patient information, in addition to links to training materials.

After the first break of the workshop, the team discusses the metrics and analytics that they will collect as part of CPOE. The team defines metrics as the measurement of how the end-users actually use the CPOE tools such as specific orders/order sets down to the provider level. We define analytics as the baseline to post-CPOE comparisons related to patient care, such as physicians' compliance to clinical pathways and improved outcomes. At their first CPOE pilots, AHS specifically measured changes in adverse drug events that cause harm and on turn-around time for Stat laboratory tests and imaging studies (pre and post-CPOE).

We then review the CPOE governance model as we discussed in Chap. 2. We feel it is important to understand how the organization makes decisions about CPOE in addition to the escalation and issue resolution processes.

Our workshop then focuses on the CPOE roadmap, with a look at the overall timeline for the facility. We use the diagram (Fig. 6.6) below as an example.

At AHS, the team used this diagram to demonstrate that the CRA helps to determine the facility's readiness to proceed with its CPOE Kick-off event. In addition, we intentionally started the CRA at our largest hospital earlier, in order to create a very engaged group of physician champions. As shown above, the major milestone of the CRA is to prepare the organization for a successful Kick-off event. Once Kick-off occurs, it is only four and one-half months until CPOE is live at the facility. This diagram creates the "burning platform" (i.e. the urgency) the leadership needs to understand to mobilize their employees and medical staff to prepare for the CPOE activation.

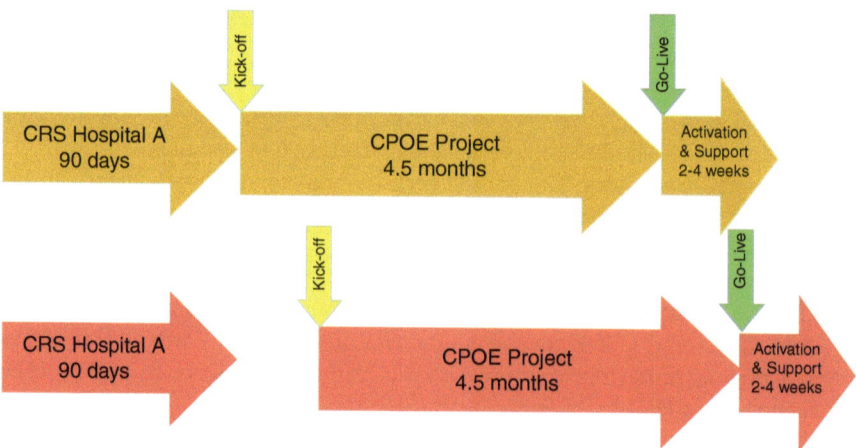

Fig. 6.6 CPOE activation snapshot. Note that the 90-day CRA determines if the facility is ready to move forward with its CPOE kickoff event

The author also like to stress that the end-point of the CPOE process is not the day of activation. Once the facility is live on CPOE, we spend the next 2–4 weeks stabilizing their processes. Once we achieve stabilization, we then focus on a more collaborative model to optimize the workflows, the providers' use of system and of our evidence-based content, and ultimately realize the benefits that we set out to achieve, related to patient safety, efficiency and effectiveness.

Drilling down further, to the next 60 days, the change manager may state the key events of the CRA processes (Table 6.1):

We discuss each of these activities above (see Chap. 5 for specifics on Leadership Interviews (Sect. 5.5) and Other Change Management Activities). One should also show how all the project threads overlap during the course of the engagement. The team can then conclude their timeline discussion with a list of major milestones, including the CRA events, key training dates, the Go/No Go decision date (About 10 days prior to activation date), and the CPOE Activation date. Then everyone takes a break.

6.2 CRA Change Management Activities

Following the break, the Change Manager facilitates the next hour of the meeting. She begins with an exercise of asking everyone to "get up and move to a different seat" (and no other instructions). After everyone has found a chair, she asks some specific questions to group and facilitates individual comments:

- "Who moved the farthest? Why?"
- "Who stayed in their seat? Why?"

Table 6.1 Key events during the CRA

CRA events	Time frame
CRA Workshop	Today
Leadership Interviews	Today and tomorrow
Denison Survey of Organizational Culture	Next week
Other Change Management Activities:	Next 60 days
Learning Assessment	
Communication Plan	
Begin Workflow Assessment	
Stakeholder Analysis	
Coaching and Retention Plans	
Board Education	
Initial MEC Meeting	

- "Why did you move where you did?"
- "Anyone not change seats? Why?"

The spontaneous answers allow the group to identify some of the common behaviors and thoughts that we experience as we face change. Some of the common answers they give are:

- "I like the opportunity to change."
- "I like to stay where I'm at."
- "You didn't give me enough directions."
- "I didn't know I could take any seat."
- "The lighting is better on this side of the room."

Then the Change Manager asks them to move again. As they all find a seat, she asks questions again, such as "What did you do this time and why?" She then asks them to return to whatever seat they desire, noting that many return to their original seat.

She then summarizes the exercise with an observation and a question. "We experienced some of the behaviors and thinking that accompany change. All we did was change our seats. Imagine what we will experience when we do CPOE!"

Moving to her formal presentation, the Change Manager defines what change management is and what it is not. She then describes our concept of a change management team within the CPOE project to connect the executives, directors, managers; project team and IT team, and help them to navigate change successfully through the project. She specifically spells out the role of the senior leaders during the CPOE project:

- To participate actively and visibly throughout the project
- To build the necessary coalition of sponsorship with the directors, managers and physician leaders/influencers
- To effectively communicate positive messages about CPOE to everyone, everyday

- To communicate commitment to success ("failure is not an option")
- To remove any barriers/obstacles

She then asks the group to think of some projects they have done and asks the question, "When we do not manage change effectively, what can we expect?" Not only do the participants benefit from processing this question. The dynamics of the room help to reveal much about the leadership team: how well do they problem-solve, share, reveal risks or collaborate; who dominates the discussion; and how much energy do they draw from each other during the participation. She summarizes the answers by reviewing some of the typical answers, as we have listed in Chap. 5.

She then revisits the project timeline in regards to the major elements/objectives relating to change. During the first 90 days, not only is the team participating in the CPOE Change Readiness Assessment, but also, they are completing Stakeholder Identification, Learning Assessment, Employee Engagement and Retention Plan, and forming a Communication Strategy and Plan. As the project kicks off, all these plans come together for continuous activities that they execute throughout the timeline. During this segment, she introduces some specific change management tools that we discussed in Chap. 5:

- The Knowledge Library (website; see *CPOE 511* in Chap. 5 as an example)
- Stakeholder Analysis
- Stakeholder Engagement Plan
- Communication Assessment
- Communication Plan, including Pulse Surveys
- Workflow Assessment and Redesign
- Employee Impact and some examples of Focus Groups
- Learning Assessment
- Training Plan
- *Denison Organizational Culture Survey* (discussed in Sect. 6.3)
- Employee Retention Plan

From there, the group moves into the next change management activity, as they review the roles and responsibilities of the Change Management Champions (see Appendix A) for the project and select appropriate leaders for each. As discussed in detail in Chap. 5, the champions are as follows:

- Stakeholder Engagement
- Communication
- Training
- Workflow
- Performance Management
- Employee Impact and Retention
- Knowledge Management
- Executive and Leadership Coaching

- Patient/Community Engagement
- Physician Engagement

It is very important that the facility assign the correct person to each role. Most of these champions must work across all levels and departments during the course of the CPOE project. Therefore, they must each have the authority and experience to lead others through their respective tasks and responsibilities. Failing to do this, the leadership team will often have to replace the champion, and thus put the success of the project at risk. The author also has found that the informatics team members should not serve as specific champions, but rather be consultative to all the various teams. Their specific expertise aids each group and they are valuable contributors to resolving operational, workflow and project issues during the course of the project.

When facilities have decided to override the CPOE team's recommendation and assign the clinical informatics or IT leads as change management champions, we have seen more stress and resistance than at other sites. In addition, replacing a champion during the project usually has significant implications, for it typically occurs once significant resistance is present as the team experiences unsuccessful management of the change process. Moreover, the clinical informatics and IT leaders tend to have a good sense for monitoring change among the end-users and recognizing when resistance is rising and enthusiasm waning.

To help the participants determine the best leaders to assign to each area, one asks them to review the criteria, roles and responsibilities for each role as we listed in Appendix A. Then one asks them to suggest names for each. Throughout the process, one should display the names of the champions either on a white board, flip chart, or through projector and fill in their recommendations. The author does not permit any one person to serve as more than one champion. In addition, he ensures that each champion either is an executive, or has an executive backing the champion up. This executive backup could be the person over the director or an executive more suited to supervise that aspect of change. Regardless, it is critical to have executive accountability and visibility for each role. The participant's selection of CPOE Champions is usually the longest exercise of the entire Executive CRA Workshop. Again, this exercise allows the CPOE leadership team presenting the workshop to observe and better understand the leadership dynamics of the hospital team. How well do they collaborate? Do they listen to each other? Who contributes and who remains silent? Is it safe to disagree? How do they resolve conflict or disagreement? How do they reach consensus or come to agreement? Their observations will provide useful insights for how the leadership currently functions as a team.

A physician on the CPOE team typically presents the next segment and last exercise of the workshop – physician engagement. We open this segment with a discussion of the five W's and the H – "What are the Who, What, When, Where, Why and How of physician engagement during a CPOE Project?" Based on the scope of the project, the presenter should answer these questions and provide a high-level overview of physician impact, disruption, and opportunities. The speaker also covers the key processes of physician engagement based on the project timeline. For example, what should they do now, what happens up until go live, and what happens after CPOE Go-live?

The exercise the presenter leads asks them to identify the names of specific members of the medical staff are in some pre-selected stakeholder groups:

- Who are the high-influencers of the medical staff?
    - These are the doctors who speak at the medical staff meetings and everyone else listens
- Who performs the most inpatient care at the hospital by volume?
- Who performs the most inpatient care at the hospital by revenue?
- Who are the physicians you see as champions for CPOE?
- Who are the physicians you see as "technology-savvy?"
- Who are the physicians who trained in hospitals with EMRs with CPOE?
- Who are the physicians who you suspect will be the most resistant to adopting CPOE?

The specific intent of this exercise is to begin the process of identifying members of key stakeholder groups. Moreover we want to observe the hospital leadership's knowledge of the medical staff as well as their team processes for collaboration and communication.

The participants typically ask many questions during this presentation and exercise. The speaker should attempt to keep the answers at a high-level and not get lost in the details (or as we like to say, keep it at 40,000 ft and keep it out of the weeds.). This is not the time to get down into every minute detail.

When the speaker has completed the exercise and answered all their questions, he ends with a final statement to make an important point, "Everything that applies for physicians holds for every employee in this hospital!"

The lead presenter closes the workshop with five critical success factors and a summary of next steps. For the AHS CPOE project, we stated the following critical success factors:

1. Know the value for patients, physicians and staff. If you cannot express it ("What's in it for me?"), then do not start yet.
2. Improve the workflow. If you cannot get physicians rounding times shorter, you have not designed a sustainable product.
3. Leadership committed, no matter what. This is not a "try-it and see" effort.
4. Know what you are trying to achieve, measure your baselines, and improve until you meet your goals. If your end state does not achieve something great, then why are you doing it?
5. Build on a solid foundation: IT, content, and the resources to be successful. You should especially have an engaged Physician Champion and excellent physician and end-user support infrastructure

We then summarize "What to do now in the C-Suite." We list out activities for each executive, reminding them that they play a critical role in the success of the

CPOE project. The final tasks for the executives are to review their calendar for competing priorities that may compete with the CPOE project and to make CPOE their major hospital initiative for a season. In addition, we give them three key points to remember:

1. Almost everything in your hospital begins with a physician order. Therefore, changing the way physicians order, changes everything.
2. While technology plays a role, CPOE is really about how well your facility handles change.
3. CPOE represents a tremendous opportunity to improve patient safety, operational outcomes and gain new efficiencies - but they do not happen by accident.

As with all CPOE events, we close with a summary slide of "the next 30 days." This will include the management team's completion of the Denison Survey online, the leadership interviews which begin that day, as well as the internal review of the information that the team obtains through survey, interviews and observations. The CPOE Leadership Team will introduce the CPOE project and review the Denison survey with the management team at their meeting near the end of those 30 days.

6.3   The Denison Organizational Culture Survey

As Dr. Jeff Rose, author and mentor to this author likes to say, "Culture eats strategy for lunch!"[4] After over a decade of doing CPOE projects, the author would like to introduce the reader to a tool that he has leveraged at over three dozen hospitals for the initial CPOE Readiness Assessments. The *Denison Organizational Culture Survey*[5] measures four traits of an organization and compares them to Denison's database of over 1,000 companies. The survey consists of 60 questions and is quite simple to administer online. We have the Chief Executive Officer (CEO) or executive sponsor send out the survey link to the entire management team of the hospital. The author only allows 1 business week for completion. The author really likes that the surveys are anonymous though we have each participant designate their leadership level (executive, director, manager or physician), and whether they classify themselves as clinical or non-clinical. We typically exceed 95 % participation in this manner.

The Denison Survey is designed to assess Mission (strategic direction and intent, goals and objectives, and vision), Consistency (core values, agreement, and coordination and integration), Adaptability (organizational learning, customer focus, and creating change), and Involvement (empowerment, team orientation, and capability development). We have found it extremely valuable in these areas of assessing organizations. One can review numerous case studies on the Denison Consulting website

---

[4] Anonymous citation, but in the CPOE world, a frequent quote of Dr. Rose.
[5] www.denisonconsulting.com.

from major companies and institutions, including one citing this author and Carlyle Walton, a hospital CEO for the Adventist Health System, who took two hospitals through successful CPOE implementations.[6]

In helping assess each hospital's management team for CPOE readiness, the CPOE team at some sites have added several custom questions to the Survey:

1. "What in your role here keeps you awake at night?"
2. "Is the organization headed in the right direction?"
3. "Would you want to be a patient here?"

In addition, the team asks them to rank the hospital's major service lines with the following two questions:

1. "What is the hospital's best service line?"
2. "Which service line do you feel has the best opportunity for improvement?"

AHS has found through the years that hospital management teams are extremely transparent and honest to their answers on our custom questions.

Denison tabulates the results and presents each organization's data back using a proprietary diagram that compares the organization against the Denison Model for their clients. The CPOE team then presents the Denison Survey directly back to the management teams in an open meeting as described in Chap. 5. The leadership teams always seem very open and appreciative as we present and validate their survey results. In addition, the custom questions have allowed these teams to shine a light on issues at each facility that may be major concerns, yet not a current focus of that organization. Through the years we have been able to use the *Denison Survey* to build on each facility's cultural strengths (e.g. Adventist Health System hospitals tend to be top decile (top 10 %) in Mission and Consistency) while helping them mitigate any risks in other areas. The author has also used the survey to help us understand the culture of hospitals as two systems merge.

The author has enjoyed a wonderful partnership with Denison. They provide third-party validation of our observations and findings and allow him to focus on other aspects of change through our CPOE projects. In addition, the leadership teams to enjoy the reports and readily validate the results. It is always useful to have a tool that gives your team, not only credibility, but reliable information, which you can leverage for your CPOE project success (Fig. 6.7).

6.4 Examples of Organizational Culture

Through the years, the author has worked with many leadership teams as they prepared for their CPOE readiness assessment. A few examples may help the reader better understand how to use the Denison Organizational Culture Survey in the process.

---

[6] Smith PA. Change readiness at Adventist Health System: how organizational culture can help hospitals implement CPOE successfully. Denison Case Stud. 2010;5:2. http://www.denisoncon-sulting.com/Libraries/Resources/Adventist_cs_201007.sflb.ashx.

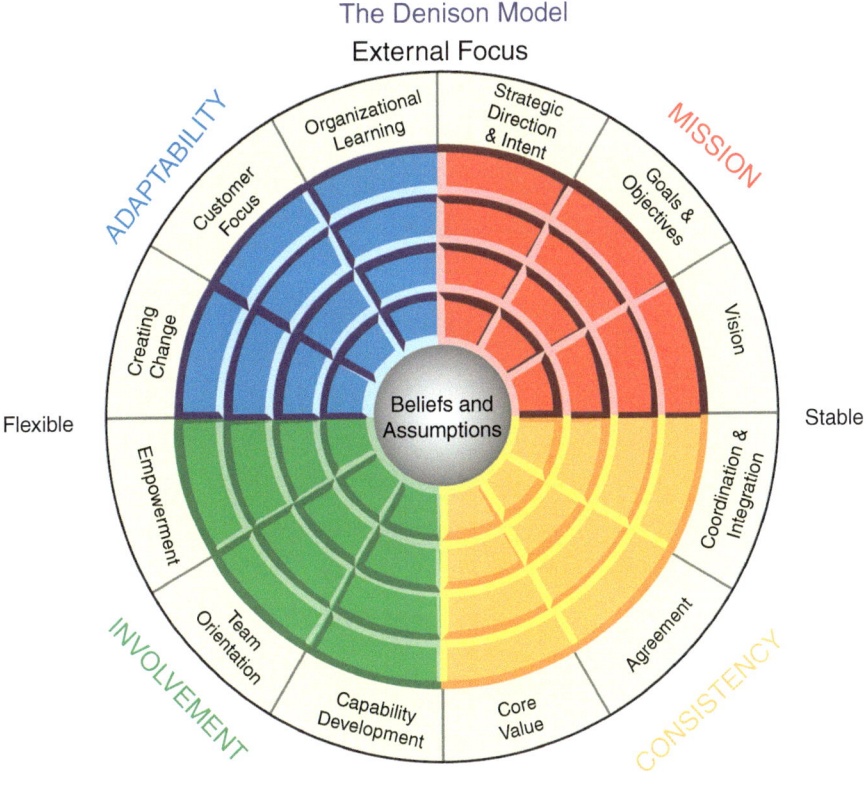

Fig. 6.7 Denison Consulting Organizational Culture Survey model (Used by permission of Denison Consulting). Each of the four concentric *circles* represents the quartile score for the organization with the *outer circle* indicating top 25 %. We find that leadership readily understands this visual report of the survey

Example 1

This hospital's leadership team was above average on many measures with strong goals and objectives, core values, a customer focus, and agreement. However, the Denison Survey showed only an average score in coordination and integration (Fig. 6.8). Their main weakness was in capability development (12th percentile) and organizational learning (44th percentile). In the assessment of this team, the team found that they were committed to work together, yet did not have clear career paths for their employees, and had cut their training budget in prior years during hard economic times.

For a CPOE project, one should realize that we would have to help them rebuild their education and training resources. We saw this as a great opportunity to create new roles and offer incentives for those staff members who stepped up to become trainers and super users. They responded positively to the change of CPOE. They saw it as an opportunity to improve their hospital's reputation and to benefit patient

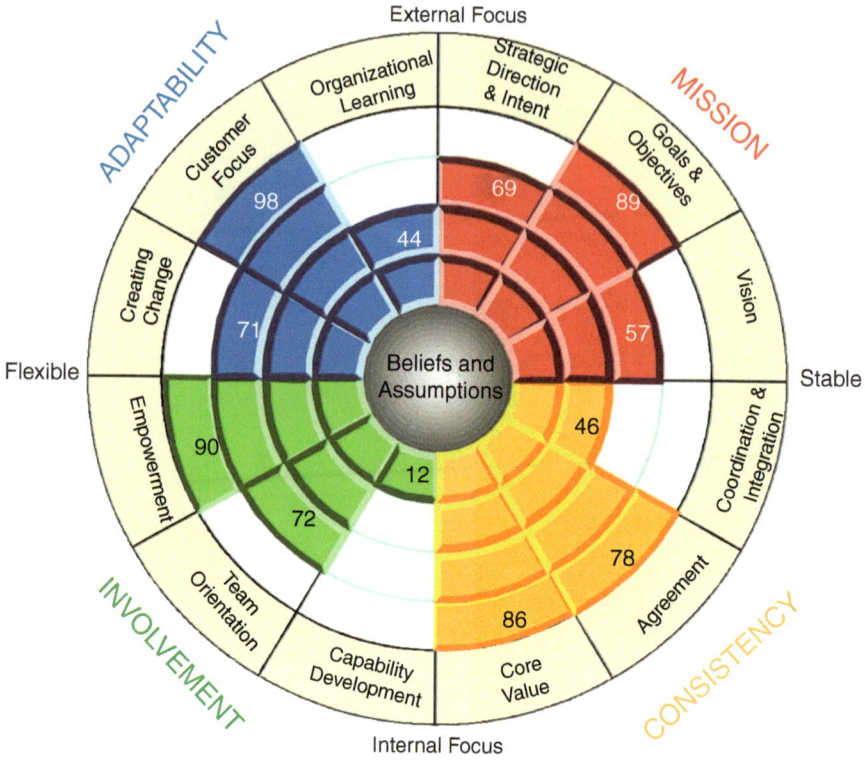

Fig. 6.8 Denison Survey of example 1

safety. Most have not had to help them define their goals and core values, but rather to embrace them throughout the project.

Example 2

The second example had a management team of 40 and was quite different from the first example (Fig. 6.9). This hospital was below average in the mission quadrant, in fact in the 15th percentile in both vision and strategic direction and intent. They had invested over a million dollars with a consulting firm over the prior 2 years to raise their customer service scores. However, with the pattern above, it is unlikely that their investment would result in any lasting change. In fact, they were bottom quartile in capability development (15th percentile), organizational learning (11th percentile) and creating change (2nd percentile). This was an organization and management team at high risk. At the time of the survey, a new executive team stepped in and successfully took this information and worked intensely on building the mission and vision of the organization. Only then were they able to take on CPOE. They experienced tremendous success with the project with less than 10 % verbal/telephone

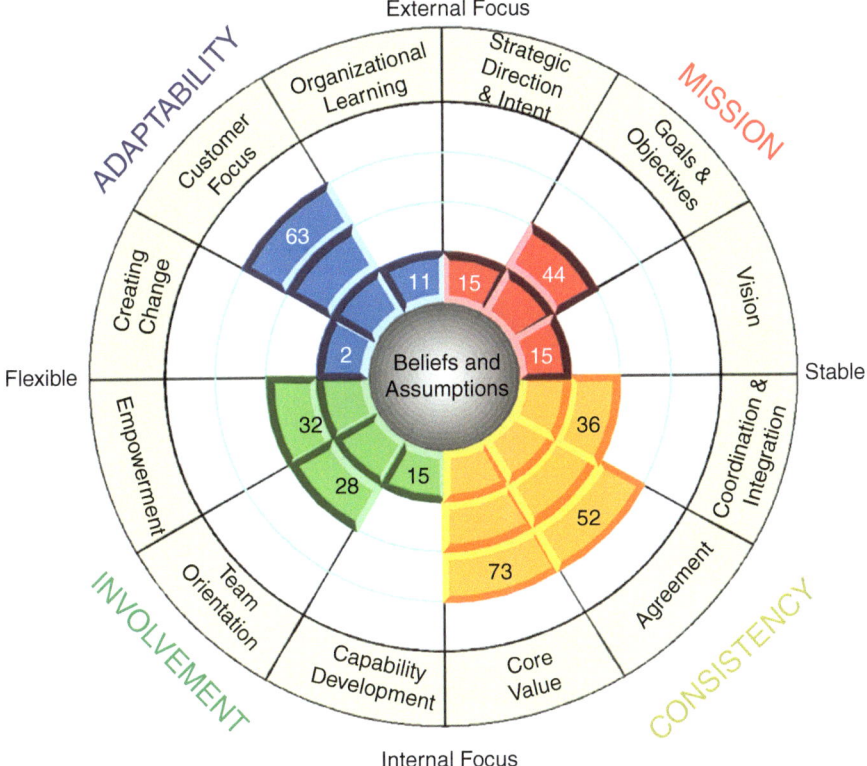

Fig. 6.9 Denison Survey for example 2

orders within days of activation. However, they did an excellent job at building their culture and engaging their management team in the process.

Example 3

This third example demonstrates the difference between the non-clinical and clinical leadership of a small health system (Fig. 6.10). While at first glance they are similar, and reflect the same organizational culture, the clinical leadership demonstrated more empowerment and a clearer sense of core values. Moreover, all three Mission scores were a quartile better for the clinicians than for the non-clinical staff.

This survey shows the influence of a strong clinical leader, despite a below average culture. Even in a stressed culture, an effective leader can rally the staff and make a difference. In a case like Example 2, it was clear to the CPOE team that the Chief Nursing Officer and the Chief Medical Officer were both strong leaders. Likewise, one should look at the non-clinical leadership for their low mission and

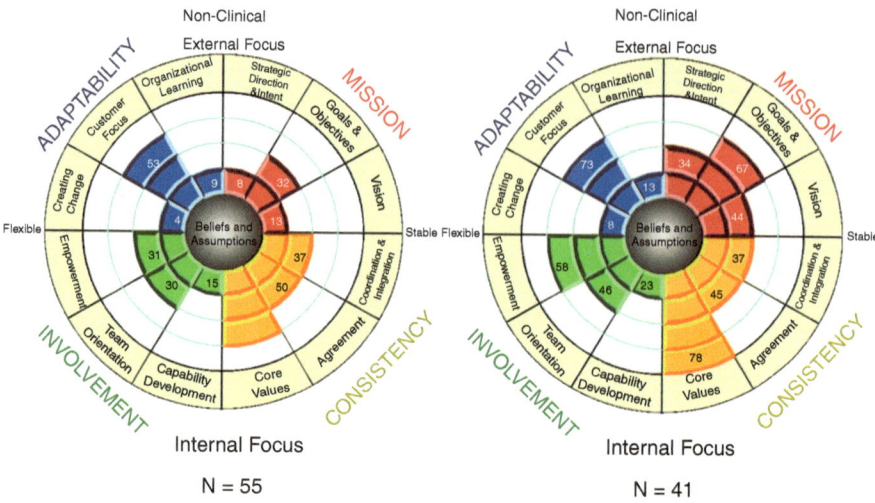

Fig. 6.10 Denison Survey for example 3

empowerment scores. This also provides some insights of the leadership over those areas. In this case, the change management strategy should include some mentoring of the non-clinical leaders, especially around their identity regarding the Mission and the empowerment of their teams. Remember that even the non-clinical employees are important to CPOE success.

In each of the three examples above, the culture was quite different and the change manager adapted the engagement plan to build on each leadership team's strengths rather than focus on their weaknesses. Moreover, not only did each leadership team come together to execute a successful CPOE project, they remained stronger after the project ended and continued to grow with future initiatives.

6.5 Key Points

- CPOE is a major change initiative. Having executive leadership on board early will reduce risks to the project
- Champions for change initiatives should be from the highest levels in the organization
- Clinical informatics and IT leadership play important consultative roles to the Champions during your CPOE project
- You can use specific exercises to help the hospital's leadership to learn to embrace and manage change
- A facility can utilize the *Denison Organizational Culture Survey* to better understand and manage their culture during a major change initiative such as CPOE

6.6 Fingernails on the Chalkboard

- **The organization has no plan to assess readiness for CPOE**
  Many organizations assume they are healthier than they really are. In addition, every group has its strengths as well as opportunities to improve. Assessing change readiness at the start of a CPOE project allows the leadership team to appreciate their current strengths and recognize where they need to put forth opportunities to improve.
- **The organization plans for IT and clinical informatics to run their CPOE project**
  While many IT and clinical informatics resources have excellent knowledge and skills in the area of change management, they often lack the organizational authority and influence to enforce major inter- and intradepartmental process changes in other hospital departments. We recommend that these team members serve in a consultative role to the change management champions during the CPOE project. They should focus themselves on system readiness and collaborate with the various champions on areas such as workflow and training, rather than having a champion role themselves.
- **The CEO is not participating with CPOE preparedness**
  CPOE affects almost every person and process in a hospital and the CEO should be the biggest supporter of a CPOE initiative. Two things happen when the CEO is not in the loop and participating on an active level. First, other major initiatives tend to appear that compete for CPOE resources. Secondly, the leadership team receives the message that CPOE is not a high priority. Therefore, these leaders have little motivation to adopt new workflow or procedures.
- **Multiple major initiatives are competing for CPOE resources**
  In that CPOE is a major initiative for a hospital, it is important that the executive team focus its undivided attention on the process. Too many major projects will dilute the resources available to manage this major change and minimize the importance of CPOE to the Medical Staff and end-users.
- **"We have a good culture," is the common assumption, so the facility chooses not to assess readiness**
  We have encountered many leadership teams that have a "culture of silence" around issues that have persisted for years. Hidden agendas and subcultures can easily derail a major initiative such as CPOE. It is far better to identify such risks early in the process and develop an approach that will help the organization to leverage its strengths while minimizing any areas of conflict or weakness.

Chapter 7
Building Momentum

Abstract This chapter discusses the specifics of how one engages the medical staff as well as the employees during the CPOE project. He discusses the hospital's formation of a Physician Informatics Committee and their role in the project. He also presents recommendations for physician and staff training, including his suggestions for each major specialty. He also suggests specific formats for key engagement events during the course of CPOE.

> Success requires first expending ten units of effort to produce
> one unit of results. Your momentum will then produce ten units
> of results with each unit of effort.[1]
> – Charles J. Givens, American Businessman

Once the organization has a defined plan for their CPOE project, is becomes time to engage the physicians and staff to build momentum toward an eventual go live date. There are many ways that an organization can engage physicians and end-users. However, this chapter presents some key steps that help to ease the process for executives, project team and the medical staff. The key of physician engagement is to lead them through the change in a systematic manner that begins with you communicating the vision, selling how CPOE will help achieve the vision, and finally, how the project affects the physician and other end-users.

As stated previously, the executive team should be fully committed to the project and the outcomes prior to embarking on physician engagement. This ensures that one or two members of the medical staff cannot individually oppose CPOE and sway the heart of one or more executives on the merits of keeping the status quo. Therefore, early in the process, we educate the leadership team and a few key physician executives on what to expect and how to overcome any objections.

During the first 90 days of the project (CPOE Readiness Assessment), the leadership should present CPOE to two important audiences. The first would be entitled

---

[1] Givens CJ. BrainyQuote.com. Retrieved from. BrainyQuote.com. Web site: http://www.brainyquote.com/quotes/quotes/c/charlesjg154638.html. Accessed 5 Feb 2012.

P.A. Smith, *Making Computerized Provider Order Entry Work*,
Health Information Technology Standards,
DOI 10.1007/978-1-4471-4243-0_7, © Springer-Verlag London 2013

"Board Education," and covers the vision, general timelines and the expected outcomes of the initiative. The presenter should be a physician who is compelling with the topic and equipped to answer the questions that will arise. Though two or three physicians typically sit on the Board, the speaker covers the subject in a manner that the lay members (i.e. members who are neither physicians nor healthcare executives) of the Board will fully understand. The presentation should be about 15 min long with 10 min additionally to answer questions. The presenter may want to meet the physician members in advance of the Board meeting to discover their commitment to the initiative and answer their questions. The ultimate goal of the presentation is to pass a resolution of Board support for the project, including the Medical Staff's mandatory usage and training of the CPOE system. The author will commonly "entertain a motion that the Board fully supports CPOE and all the related policies and procedures including the mandatory usage and training by the medical staff." Typically, a physician on the Board will advance the motion and the Board approves unanimously. Board endorsement provides important validation of the project and allows the hospital CEO to hold firm when physician resistance occurs later in the project.

7.1 Physician Engagement

The second early event should be a general medical staff meeting with an opportunity to provide continuing medical education (CME) credits to the physicians. For the last several years, the author uses a presentation called, *"The Evidence behind CPOE."* The purpose of this presentation is to provide information from peer-reviewed journals and industry experts on the rationale behind CPOE, the outcomes you should expect from CPOE and the opportunities to improve safety, efficiency and effectiveness. He recommends that you include CPOE studies that represent key articles that cite problems that have derailed CPOE project or created negative outcomes,[2] in addition to any studies that show how subsequent projects have mitigated such risks.[3] It is then up to the presenter to demonstrate how the current CPOE project has ensured a safer product. The rationale of the CME meeting is achieving several objectives for your project:

• Build a strong evidence-based case for CPOE
• Introduce articles which place a cloud over CPOE, and have open discussion on how you plan to mitigate these risks

---

[2] Watson S, Nguyen TC, et al. Unexpected increased mortality after implementation of a commercially sold computerized physician order entry system. Pediatrics. 2005;116:1506.
[3] Longhurst CA, Parast L, et al. Decrease in hospital-wide mortality rate after implementation of a commercially sold computerized physician order entry system. Pediatrics. 2010;126:14.

- Provide the physicians with a town-hall experience in which you first educate them, then directly respond to their questions
- Take a pulse of the medical staff on attitudes and resistance toward CPOE

Moreover, if the organization has internal data supporting CPOE, the presenter should include that as well. These meetings typically are quite helpful and energizing. However, you may also have some members of the medical staff confront you, or become active resisters of the process. For the faint of heart, the author should remind the presenter, "What does not kill you only makes you stronger."[4] In addition, the presenter should not use this initial meeting to demonstrate software or specific physician workflow. It is important that the presenter keep the crowd at a high level, and firmly establish the business case for CPOE at the hospital.

This is your first meeting to drive the vision of the project to the medical staff. The author specifically recommends that this initial meeting **not** be a demonstration of CPOE or the software. Diving into specific clicks and screens will dilute the message of the vision for your project. There will be specific opportunities for you to have these demonstrations and discussions when it will be most effective. To put it another way, this meeting is about the "why" of CPOE and not about the "how."

If the hospital does not have a physician executive, such as Vice President of Medical Affairs, Chief Medical Officer, or Chief Medical Information Officer on its team, it is important that the hospital identify a physician to provide oversight to the local project needs. Typically, this physician will be a local member of the medical staff who has an interest in safety, quality or informatics. Recognizing that not every hospital has a full time physician executive, the hospital should budget at least 17 h/month for this role and arrange for that physician to commit to full time help beginning with the onset of CPOE training through the go live and at least 2 weeks thereafter. Thereafter, the physician should be available to support medical peers up to half time (10–20 h/week) for 2 months. In most cases, the hospital will contract with the physician for this time (i.e. pay), or hire outright. If multiple hospitals are involved, we recommend a uniform rate for physician time, as long as salary surveys support your rate. Likewise, the hospital should identify four to six key physicians to serve as physician champions for CPOE. These physicians should represent a cross section of the medical staff and serve as charter members of your Physician Informatics Committee (keeping it bigger than CPOE alone), which the author will discuss further below. He recommends that you include at least one high-risk physician on this committee. An example would be the doctor who passionately speaks at every medical staff meeting, but always with a hint of insight and truth. This doctor will then be an insider to your project, provide unfiltered feedback, and ultimately have "skin in the game" when you do go live with CPOE. In addition, avoid putting only technically competent physicians on the committee.

---

[4] Friedrich Nietzsche.

Another model the author has used successfully is to contract for a physician in each major specialty who represent their peer group, learn the CPOE workflow and own training of the medical staff. These physician trainer-champions typically commit 2 h monthly for presentations and exposure to CPOE techniques and processes, complete 4–8 h of training, then actually teach classes for their specialty. Of course, the hospital contracts with these physicians in advance and reimburse them for their time. In teaching hospitals, this previously became a moonlighting opportunity. This practice now has become more challenging with work hours limitations on residents. AHS has used the physician trainer-champion model in a hospital very successfully with a medical staff in excess of 700. The physicians divided the medical staff roster and each took accountability for 30–40 physicians. They trained them with a defined syllabus which they themselves then practiced on their own and used with their own classes. Not only did the 20 trainer-champions take their roles very seriously and deliver first-class instruction, but also they represented a solid group of super-users at go-live. The peer-to-peer classroom interactions were superb without the typical distractions and debates of other methods.

As noted above, the local physician executive should work with the Chief of Staff to establish a Physician Informatics Committee (PIC), subcommittee or group. This group meets monthly, and become true insiders to the CPOE project (as well as future initiatives). The PIC serves several key functions:

- The project physician (CMIO or Medical Director) trains each member of the PIC on the CPOE workflows early in the project and provides answers to common questions as well as techniques to overcome resistance,
- The PIC provides regular updates on the CPOE project to the Medical Executive Committee and at other meetings of the medical staff,
- The PIC physicians promote CPOE to their peers from a position of knowledge of the evidence for CPOE and their personal experience through training,
- The PIC provides a structure for reviewing evidence-based order sets, clinical decision support rules and other content,
- The PIC becomes the sounding board for the medical staff after go live, and
- The PIC keeps key physicians as a focus group for new EMR initiatives.

A hospital with an active PIC has a wonderful resource behind their CPOE project.

The Project Kickoff also becomes a tremendous opportunity to engage members of the medical staff. Like most events during CPOE, the Kickoff should be a town hall format, allowing participants to ask questions and get answers in a group setting. The author discusses this event in detail, below, under Staff Engagement.

He recommends that the next two physician events occur 1 and 2 months prior to the onset of CPOE physician training. The theme of these two events is "A Day in the Life of the Physician." At AHS, we called these events "CPOE Sneak Peak 1" and "Sneak Peak 2" and gave them a movie premiere theme. The organizer of these events should carefully review the scope of the project and present a multi-disciplinary story of how the physician performs common workflows once CPOE goes live.

The author recommends the first story focus on several care scenarios the patient may experience through the hospital stay:

- The patient presenting to the Emergency Department,
- The healthcare team's delivery of care within the ED,
- The admission process to a critical care unit,
- The transfer process to a medical/surgical nursing unit, and
- The physician discharge process.

Throughout the story, the presenter(s) highlight the how CPOE communicates orders immediately to nurses, lab and the imaging department, and the positive impact to patient care and safety. The author strongly recommends that this presentation include screenshots from the EMR rather than live code, so the presenter can more quickly and succinctly through the content in about 15–20 min, leaving 10–15 min for the audience's questions. It is important to remember that the primary goal is help the physicians get answers to their questions and to begin to see how it all comes together. This is not an opportunity to perform a deep-dive into the EMR. The team should answer any questions that physicians raise as well as posting them on the FAQ site.

The second day-in-life of a physician event has the team present other workflows that will help the physicians obtain a clearer picture of their workflow. One often covers physician documentation, rules and alerts, and medical records processes within the EMR. Again, the presenter should leave plenty of time for the physicians to understand the workflows and ask questions. Potential topics include:

- Medical records management (co-signing orders, documents)
- Messaging
- Clinical decision support (CDS, rules and alerts)
- Physician electronic documentation
- And other topics in scope not covered in the prior event

You should have sign-in sheets for both of these events. These two group events typically draw good numbers, and if not, indicate that your Communication Plan may not be effective.

7.2 Physician Training

Through the years, the author has seen a wide spectrum of techniques, tools and timings on this subject. One must consider the scope of the CPOE project and the current state of the end users in use of the EMR. In addition, there may be resource constraints, competing projects and momentum considerations. However, there are logical steps you can take to develop a plan for success. Project management principles of scope, resources and timeline, are valuable tools in this process. One should begin with a training champion, the director or vice president that the organization assigns accountability for a successful CPOE training plan and execution.

Starting with scope, the project manager, training champion and workflow champion should answer the following questions:

- What functionality will be new in the EMR when we activate CPOE?

    – Of this functionality, what will affect physician workflow?

- How do physicians interact with the EMR today prior to CPOE?

    – Do they mainly view the chart?
    – Do they personally enter data/information during patient care?
    – Do they manage HIM (health information management, or medical records completion) workflow (such as electronically signing dictated/transcribed documents) in the EMR today?
    – Do they perform physician documentation in the EMR today?
    – Do they enter and maintain Problem Lists within the EMR?
    – Do they use secure messaging to other users within the EMR?
    – What results/reports (e.g. lab results, imaging reports or transcribed documents) do the hospital employees print for doctors today from the EMR even though they are available for viewing within the electronic chart?

- Do physicians use the EMR remotely (at home or office)?

    – How do physicians log in to the EMR remotely and in hospital?
    – Does this remote access allow physicians to do CPOE or only viewing?

- What are physicians' general attitudes toward the current EMR and toward CPOE?
- What will be the physicians' responsibility and workflow with CPOE (i.e. the physician's future state)?

    – In what venues of care will the doctor use CPOE or remain on paper?
    – Is electronic physician documentation in scope?
    – Will physicians enter and maintain an electronic Problem List?
    – How will clinical decision support affect the physicians, such as alerts, rules, embedded reminders or evidence-based order sets?
    – How will physicians provide feedback on CPOE content?
    – How will the organization communicate future changes to the physicians once CPOE is live?
    – How will the organization keep evidence-based order sets up to date?
    – What are the downtime procedures?
    – How does the hospital train new members of the medical staff?

In addition to these specific questions, the training and workflow champions will need a complete understanding of the vision of the project (see Chap. 1) as well as the specific CPOE policies and procedures (see Chap. 2). The author really likes to stress the difference between physician decision-making (i.e. medical decision-making) and nursing decision-making (also known as clinical decision-making). Prior to CPOE, one realizes that many hospitals and medical staffs have blurred those two processes. CPOE becomes a great opportunity to separate the two with clear processes and accountabilities.

The discharge process is an important interdisciplinary workflow to include in CPOE. The key stakeholders in this process are the physician, the nurse, the patient, the patient's family/caregiver and the registration clerk. It is important that each stakeholder knows his responsibilities and workflows for his piece of the larger process.

The physician is responsible for medical decision-making. This includes the decision to discharge and the medical discharge plan. The physician must write an order for discharge, and then have all the other medical-decision steps in his workflow. These decisions are similar with most patients:

- Is it an appropriate time to discharge the patient?
- Where is the patient going after discharge?
- If not going home, has the receiving facility accepted the patient?
- If going home, does the patient need in-home health services and are they scheduled?
- What medications should the patient take following hospital discharge? The physician accomplishes this through discharge medication reconciliation.
- What new prescriptions does the patient need and how should we communicate them (i.e. printed, called to pharmacy or electronically transmitted)?
- What diet, activities and restrictions should the patient follow?
- What education materials should accompany the patient home regarding the primary diagnosis and/or procedures relating to the hospital stay?
- Which physicians will the patient follow up with after discharge and when?
- Are any supplies (i.e. durable medical equipment or DME) the patient needs for home care?

Ideally, the physician should own these decisions and indicate them directly into the EMR. These orders and documentation should flow automatically onto the patient's discharge instructions, be expressed in patient language and not medical-speak, and not require anyone else to transcribe the information elsewhere. The physician also completes a summary of care document (e.g. a discharge summary) to finalize the medical record.

The nurse has four primary responsibilities in the discharge process:

- The return of any valuables to the patient
- The review of the discharge plan with the patient/caregiver to ensure that complete comprehension occurs (i.e. ensure medical literacy of the patient for his discharge instructions)
- The nurse obtains the patient's sign-off of the instructions and provides them in the patient's preferred media (i.e. printed, on electronic media, or by secure messaging)
- The nurse communicates to the transport team to assist in the physical discharge of the patient from the facility then notifies registration that the patient is leaving

The patient typically is responsible for transportation home with appropriate friends or family to accompany him. The patient is also responsible for his understanding and follow-up of the medical discharge plan.

Prior to CPOE, one often sees confusion of these roles around the discharge process. With a seamless discharge process, the author has witnessed a 4–6 h discharge process shrink to a 15–30 min process. This reengineering should result in a more efficient process and higher patient satisfaction, as family members no longer wait hours until the "paperwork is done."

In the early planning of the project, the training champion should inventory the available training space and capacity. The inventory includes the layout and number of computers in each classroom, the number of classrooms, as well as the location of the classrooms. The training champion uses this information for determining the logistical plan of training of all users, not only the physicians. However, the training champion should assess whether there are any physical or location barriers that impede physicians (or staff) from attending training (such as expecting them to travel 20 miles to a training facility on their own time.). The author recommends that each classroom facilitate training 12–16 users, have plenty of room for proctors to move among (specifically behind) the trainees, and have at least one LCD projector. If a second LCD projector is available, the instructor may use that to project the training agenda and/or key points.

The author's ideal training room is U-shaped so that all participants can see each other rather than each other's monitor. As the participants arrive, the instructor is looking for the person who might be most anxious of the class. That participant, one should ask to sit at the bottom of the U, facing the top of the U, and projecting his training computer (via the LCD projector) onto the front wall.

Personally, the author trains with this end-user in the driver's seat and the author glancing intermittently at the screen to make sure the person is keeping up with the workflow. In addition, he is paying attention to the training agenda and the trainees.

There are proctors roaming behind the trainees to assist and ensure that each is keeping on task. Ideally, you would like to have one proctor for every three to four trainees. The author also prefers physician proctors to be super users from the department relevant to the physician. For example, a surgical super user would proctor classes for surgeons and anesthesiologists while an obstetrical nurse super user might proctor classes for obstetricians and for pediatricians.

The author's psychology with this technique is that the class sees a peer navigating the chart. This also prevents the instructor from moving too fast, especially if he knows the system well. In addition, he can best interact with the participants as he moves around the center of the room and maintains eye contact.

Once the training champion completes the inventory of the physical space, she must ascertain the number of end-users she must train. One might like to divide classes so that the main groups can train on their specific workflows:

- Primary Care Specialties and Medical Hospitalists

  - Admitting a patient, including admission medication reconciliation and the registration order
  - Direct admissions from the office to hospital
  - Transferring a patient from one level of service to another, including transfer medication reconciliation
  - Discharge process, including discharge order, discharge medication reconciliation, writing/e-prescribing new prescriptions as well as durable medical equipment (e.g. oxygen, walkers), patient instructions (diet, activity, wound care, etc.), follow-up with physicians after discharge and in-home services
  - Daily rounds with progress note and orders
  - Management of inbox, such as signing verbal/telephone orders and documents

- Surgeons

  - Admitting a patient, including admission medication reconciliation and the registration order
  - Transferring a patient from one level of service to another, including transfer medication reconciliation
  - Discharge process, including discharge order, discharge medication reconciliation, writing/e-prescribing new prescriptions as well as durable medical equipment (e.g. oxygen, walkers), patient instructions (diet, activity, wound care, etc.), follow-up with physicians after discharge and in-home services
  - Daily rounds with progress note and orders
  - Management of inbox, such as signing verbal/telephone orders and documents
  - Planning/placing pre-admission testing orders
  - Planning/placing pre-operative (i.e. morning of surgery) orders
  - Processes in the PACU (post-anesthesia care unit) such as electronic operative notes, intra-PACU orders (for inventions within the PACU, such as starting patient-controlled analgesia, or post operative x-rays), workflow for a patient the surgeon is discharging to home after recovery and for the patient the surgeon is admitting to the hospital for a longer stay

- Emergency Physicians

  - Emergency Department triage policies, procedures, and order sets
  - ED orders

  - ED documentation, both as single assessments and as repeated assessments
  - Intra-ED consultations
  - Admitting to hospital processes (with attention to whether the ED physician or the admitting physician enters the actual admission orders or transition orders)

- Pediatricians

  - Similar to the Primary Care Specialties above except for more training on weight-based and age-based ordering of medications
  - Familiarity with pediatric order set content

- Obstetricians

  - Similar to Surgeons above except for additional training for planning labor orders, in-hospital labor orders, vaginal delivery and Cesarean notes, and post-partum orders

- Psychiatrists

  - Similar to Primary Care Specialties above
  - Specialty notes for psychiatric care documentation
  - Familiarity with behavioral health order set content

- Radiologists and Pathologists

  - Mainly orders and the content and tools for their workflows
  - Opportunity to review navigation of the EHR so that these physicians can easily review pertinent patient information
  - Interventional Radiologists need training similar to surgeons, regarding pre-procedure and post-procedure orders

All physicians get training in basic orders, order sets and any additional tools that physicians use for CPOE. In addition, training may cover topics such as multi-modal insulin and hyperglycemia management, venous thromboembolism (VTE) prophylaxis, electrolyte replacement protocols and strategies for meeting the national inpatient quality measures.

The training champion will look at the number of physicians in each group and determines the number of classes she will offer for each group. Typically, the author likes physician classes in the morning, mid-day, and later afternoon or early evening. Many facilities choose to offer weekend and night classes as well to the medical staff.

In addition to the logistics of classroom training, the training champion needs to determine the type and duration of training to offer. We have found through the years that a combination of computer-based training (CBL, or computer-based learning) and classroom (hands-on training) create a healthy balance in knowledge transfer. Of course, one must factor in the scope of the project and the level of competency and skills the physician users currently possess. Through the years, the author has witnessed many training methods, and combination of methods, and have some observations to share on the topic.

"After 12 years of doing CPOE projects across the country, we had a wonderful laboratory with the AHS CPOE project that allowed us to validate some observations we had seen previously. At our first two CPOE sites, we were able to try variations in training methodologies and follow those physicians through the process. The variables were CBLs before classroom; CBLs after classes; no CBL, only classes; and one-on-one training versus classes.

"We found very quickly with the medical staff of these two pilot hospitals, that the doctors who transitioned best to CPOE were the ones that did CBL's prior to classes, then trained in workflow for their specialty, in group (rather than one-on-one) classes. That then became our prescribed methodology that we have asked all our hospitals to support.

"We acknowledge that other variations, such as one-on-one training, would intuitively seem superior, and many have questioned the usefulness of CBLs. However, our experience has demonstrated otherwise.

"The intent of the CBLs is to give an overview of the admission/transfer/discharge process, the purpose of CPOE, and present repeatedly some processes that physicians need to know for patient care in a CPOE environment. Therefore, when they get to class, they are familiar with the layout of the chart, the icons, and have a big picture of what they are doing. The ones that come to class without CBLs tend to drag the class down with endless agendas ("I don't know why we are doing this?" "You don't expect me to do this?" and so on) and actually disrupt those who have been compliant, done their CBLs and are there to learn hands-on. Therefore, the CBLs are like teaching arithmetic prior to algebra or calculus. Student who skip arithmetic make the learning process more difficult. We have now trained over 10,000 doctors and midlevels, in the past three years, so now have significant experience on this topic."

The CBLs also serve as a vetting process. Physicians who specifically refuse to do the prescribed training become your high-risk physicians who need an opportunity for one-on-one dialogue with the CEO or a physician peer. This one-on-one engagement allows the leader to reinforce the vision of the initiative, his commitment to the resistant physician, and the reality that the Board has prescribed mandatory training as a requirement for continued participation on the medical staff. The leader should follow up personally with the resistant physician frequently for the next several days until he completes his training. Once these resistant physicians actually complete training, they often comment that it "is better than I thought." Winning one of your resistant physicians through this process is priceless to the success of your project. It seems that the entire medical staff is aware when your resistant physician gets on board with CPOE. Likewise, if you make one exception, the entire medical staff knows that as well.[5]

The author has also observed that even one-on-one training hurts the physician over classroom training. The instructor seems to exhibit more of a rush to get the one-on-one class over, and miss the opportunity to get peers asking questions, and ensuring that the doctors are really grasping the workflows. However, sometimes the instructor must provide one-on-one training in order to catch a few of the physicians. He recommends you make one-on-one training the exception, not the norm.

The team should also ask the entire executive team to complete all the CBLs and attend at least one physician class. This helps the executive to respond with encouragement when a physician balks at completing the CBLs or attending class. Without that training, the executive becomes more sympathetic to doctors who state they are "too busy to train," or "The CBLs are worthless." The trained executive can look the physician in the eye and

---

[5] With tribute to the classic Parker Brothers game, Monopoly[TM], we call this unfortunate phenomenon, "Giving them a get-out-of-jail-free card." This is a very costly error on the part of the CEO. Every physician needs to train.

remind him that poor training on the front end will cost the physician more time in the end, due to confusion, rework, and suboptimal efficiency. Moreover, it is effective when the executive says, "I didn't find them that bad at all!"

Spending sufficient time to construct a training plan will allow the facility to build momentum leading up to go live and create a foundation on which physicians can build their efficiency and effectiveness of patient care. Not properly training physicians will ensure more conflict at go live from the doctors who are not prepared and actively complain.

7.3   Staff Engagement

While many intuitively think that physician-engagement is the key to CPOE success, the staff numbers and complexity are much greater than the size of the medical staff. The author discussed the details of the change management plan in Chaps. 5 and 6. However, they are some specific recommendations that you may find helpful.

While he has stated repeatedly that, the CEO/Executive Sponsor must lead the CPOE project; the author recommends some specific behaviors on the part of the entire management team as well. They should attend each event, showing up with enthusiasm and interest. They should not be checking email on their mobile phones or personal digital assistants, having "sidebar conversations," or be doing any other activity that demonstrates that the message/event is not important. Moreover, after the event, they should specifically engage the attendees and openly offer to answer questions. We encourage you to frame questions in a positive manner. We recommend questions like, "Do you see the opportunities we see with CPOE?" and not, "What do you think?"

Among the management team members, they are several critical success factors that we must recommend strongly:

1. As mentioned above, the entire executive team should complete the physician training curriculum, including viewing all CBLs and attending at least one physician class. This gives the executives extreme credibility when a physician refuses training and says they do not have time to train. Responses that come to mind include "Oh, I didn't find that it took me very long to complete those," "I found them helpful," or "I really have seen, through training, how this is going to make us a better hospital!" Moreover, the executives should intentionally report their training completion at the monthly Champion Meeting. The word seems to get out to all the employees and medical staff that the entire executive team has trained.
2. Likewise, every director and manager should follow the lead of the executives. They should be the first to train on their units and in their departments. Otherwise, they will not make wise decisions when their department members discuss new workflows. They should do everything possible to free up their staff to attend key CPOE events. In addition, they should hold monthly huddles on CPOE and accelerate those to weekly, once training begins. The huddles are 3–5 min conversations to reinforce

key impacts or workflow changes that the unit/department will experience once CPOE goes live. The manager/director eventually covers the Start/Stop/Continue Document during these important conversations with staff.

3. Managers should protect training time for their employees. The author has seen managers call their employees into work rather to train with no notice, or even pull the employee out of a class in process. While this is the occasional reality of running a hospital, one should raise the red flag if it happens on a frequent or recurrent basis. This may be the first sign that your manager is either not on board with employee training, or may not be very proactive in managing the human resources. Either way, the training manager should escalate cancellations to the Training Champion for further investigation, and discussion at the appropriate level within the organization.

With the above in mind, the leaders recognize that the staff will experience some fear and anxiety throughout the CPOE project. Because CPOE changes or affects almost every process in the hospital, we cannot remind leaders enough the importance of two-way communication with your staff throughout the process. There must be many opportunities for staff to ask questions and ventilate their concerns.

Throughout every day of training, the team should maintain a "parking lot list" of questions that end-users raise for which the instructor(s) do not know the answer. They should research them and recognize many of them are often workflow questions. As the training manager determines the answers to these questions and concerns, he should forward them to the Knowledge Management and Workflow champions as necessary for them to include in either the FAQ (frequently asked questions) or the appropriate Stop/Start/Continue Document. The manager should also brief the instructors daily on content changes or any new FAQ submissions.

The training team should also utilize a tracking tool of end-users and medical staff members as they complete CBLs, classroom work and practice. In addition, each end-user should complete some type of competency evaluation, which the trainers administer. The training manager should update the tracking tool weekly and report against weekly training goals. The training statistics should include overall facility training achievement as well as a breakdown to the individual units/departments. The Training Champion should report at the weekly Champion meetings during the last month leading up to activation.

7.4   Key Points

- Physician and staff engagement have key events with each event having a specific intent to accomplish
- Board education leads to early Board commitment to your CPOE project
- Lead physicians through a specific process
  - First communicate the vision
  - Help them understand your business case for CPOE

- Educate them on the benefits of CPOE to themselves and their patients
- Openly discuss the risks of CPOE and your plan to mitigate those risks
- Form a Physician Informatics Committee (PIC)
- Have specific physician leadership through champions and your PIC
- Mandate training and use of CPOE
- Do not compromise your mandates or make any exceptions

- Have the entire executive team complete the physician training program
- Have the entire management team be the first to train for CPOE
- Stress two-way communication over flyers and speeches
- Have department/unit super-users proctor physicians who typical deliver care on those units.

7.5 Fingernails on the Chalkboard

- **The CEO allows one influential or high-volume physician to continue writing orders**
  If you have made CPOE mandatory, which we highly recommend, then you will put the entire effort in jeopardy if that mandate has exceptions. It not only opens the door for other physicians, but it communicates to the hospital staff that this one doctor operates on a different set of rules than everyone else. Actions like this will breed distrust and the credibility of the executive's integrity. The CEO who holds the line when a physician challenges the hospital's resolve will usually put an end to future medical staff challenges.
- **The CEO allows one influential or high-volume physician to not complete the full training**
  When a CEO allows a physician to only partially train, the executive has opened the door for others to follow suit. Moreover, a physician who has not properly trained usually becomes frustrated with CPOE and may publicly vocalize such frustration. More importantly, though, the CEO is allowing the physician to practice medicine in the CPOE hospital with unsafe education and training. CPOE is not simple, nor without risk to the patient when a physician performs it improperly. The CEO should first examine the question "Would I allow this physician to perform an operation for which he is not trained?" This is not an issue of the intelligence or competency of the physician to perform other medical duties. CPOE is the physician's application of new technology to guide every order he writes. Once they understand this analogy, most physicians will commit to training, though their objections will persist through the implementation and weeks later.
- **A director or manager does not complete training early**
  The manager/director of the unit/department sets the entire tone for her staff. It is critical for the leader to lead by example, and this is no exception. When the leader is not the first to train, several consequences predictably occur:

1. The leader cannot effectively lead the staff through productive workflow design, or contradicts the appropriate CPOE workflow
2. The leader is less likely to free up staff time for them to attend key CPOE events
3. The team has less enthusiasm and more apathy for CPOE
4. The team expresses more resistance
5. The team does not leverage CPOE to improve workflow efficiencies and settles for doing things "the way they always have done them."
6. The team falls behind on training goals
7. The team is often ill-prepared at go live
8. The team takes months to leverage CPOE or may never achieve productivity gains or overcome resistance

- **Training progress is not transparent**
  The management team will discover several important processes that the hospital should follow during the training phase. The Training Champion should produce a sound Training Plan with clear objectives, such as the date training starts, what training looks like by stakeholder group or unit, and how do end-users schedule themselves into classes. The Training Champion must set weekly training completion goals with minimal standards for the numbers/percentages of the staff (as well as one for the medical staff). The Training Champion may publicize these goals, as well as the actual completion rates for staff and physicians by group. We recommend you track the management team as well to hold leadership accountable. At the weekly Champion meeting, the Training Champion reports out on the specific training statistics for the physicians, the staff, and if you have it, the management team. The CPOE team also uses the training completion data to make a final "Go/No Go" call about 10–14 days prior to the activation data. As you keep the training data transparent, it helps to motivate the team.
  The training champion may want to publicly recognize end-users or physicians who are the first to train. We always recommend focusing on the successes and not the resisters.
- **Few opportunities exist for two-way communication**
  The CPOE team should be looking for every opportunity to "talk-up" CPOE and create dialogue on the project and its benefits. This is not the type of project that relies on flyers, posters and emails. Those vehicles are important to announce CPOE focus groups, meeting, town halls or other events, but not to sell CPOE to the masses. Almost every person in the hospital will face some change in workflow from CPOE implementations. This means fear, doubt, resistance and sometimes even outright rebellion. Failing to plan for two-way dialogue throughout the project is a recipe for failure. In addition, we recommend that you provide food/refreshments during the key events, not just for the physician events. This is not a time to scrimp on the budget, but rather show your gracious appreciation for the work and sacrifice of the change ahead.

Chapter 8
Avoiding Common Pitfalls

Abstract This chapter presents numerous opportunities for the reader to avoid common pitfalls during a CPOE project. This begins with the author's discussion of budget assumptions and planning for the project's implementation and support. The author intends this chapter to allow the reader to avoid traps and issues common to many CPOE projects. In addition, he presents recommendations for the characteristics of the key physician support personnel and staffing guidelines. He also discusses the importance of addressing the physicians' responsibility for medical decision-making prior to CPOE implementation.

> *Criticism is something we can avoid easily by saying nothing,*
> *doing nothing, and being nothing*
>
> *– Aristotle*

Before discussing implementation in Chap. 9, it may be helpful to discuss some common pitfalls that seem to be prevalent with CPOE projects. While each Chapter's Fingernails on the Chalkboard provide some common examples of pitfalls related to the topic, the author will use this chapter to discuss opportunities that may provide some additional insights for success.

8.1 Budget Assumptions for Planning for CPOE at a Facility

The hospital leadership team should budget appropriately for the CPOE implementation. Otherwise, they will under-support the project at critical times, which will result in poor execution or in poor results. Therefore, the facility/health system should develop a model for CPOE planning and implementation.

The team can typically make the assumptions that the management team (managers, directors and senior leaders) will be "all in" for CPOE, and not result in any additional salary costs. They can also assume that there will be some permanent training,

P.A. Smith, *Making Computerized Provider Order Entry Work*,
Health Information Technology Standards,
DOI 10.1007/978-1-4471-4243-0_8, © Springer-Verlag London 2013

IT technical support, clinical informatics and physician support roles that will be permanent costs within the organization. However, it is useful to estimate additional costs that the facility will expend during course of the CPOE project. The largest expense is typically the additional hours of non-salaried employees, who often must log overtime in the process of training. Since projects may span more than one budget period, it is useful to have a model that provides estimates within the phases of the project. These estimates (including Table 8.1) do not include the IT department resources of the CMIO, clinical informatics and project management, which are typically part of the existing infrastructure of a hospital or health system. We tend to estimate the additional CPOE costs at the facility level with the following logic:

- **CPOE Readiness Assessment**: Involves all members of the executive team, pharmacy director, informatics team, HR director and key physicians. Includes Denison Survey of Organizational Culture, interviews and numerous activities to assessment your facility (people, processes and technology) and prepare for successful CPOE planning and ideal activation target date. Outside of the cost of the Denison Survey, this 90-day process has a minimal staff cost.

- **CPOE Project (Prep)**: Once the team determines the CPOE activation (go live) date, the kickoff is scheduled for 4.5 months prior. The first 3 months will continue the preparation of the medical staff and employees for CPOE, and validate workflow and content needs. Major components include the team's understanding of how each unit does its online work, compared to documented workflows for CPOE success. This includes moving staff toward complete utilization of current online EMR tools, as well as real-time documentation of vital signs, clinical assessments, and eMAR administration. Two "Sneak Peak" (also known as "Day-in-the-Life") events (which the team holds as Town Hall type of events) and bimonthly pulse surveys monitor the success of the communication plan. The team's project preparation also includes concurrent scanning, which will begin prior to CPOE activation date. A facility can clearly allocate time commitments for hourly staff for these activities.

- **CPOE Project (Training)**: This 6–8 week segment includes Train-the-Trainer, as well as end-user training of all clinical, HIM, ancillary staff as well as all physicians and pertinent office staff. Training includes online as well as in class training and practice, as well as "observed competencies" of all end-users. This is also the time that the staff and physicians really understand the impact of CPOE to their workflow and will begin to ask serious questions around specific workflows and possibly identify potential workflow issues that the team has not previously addressed during the earlier phase.

- **Activation Support**: On the morning of activation, the physicians start entering orders online, which affects almost every department and process within the hospital. Unit-based support will rely on well-trained facility Super-Users who understand all CPOE workflows, including physician and staff. While the on-unit facility support will continue for 30 days, the CPOE project team will provide additional workers. Dedicated Super-User support will be necessary for each unit/ department for the first 15 days, then scale back to roving Super-User support for the second 15 days, with the understanding that working Super-Users will still be available as first-call resources on each unit. The trained Super-Users will be

Table 8.1 Estimated facility hours for CPOE implementation (30–350 beds)

Event	Total facility (h)	Salary (h)	Non-salary (h)
CPOE readiness assessment	530	530	0
CPOE prep/planning	2,879–4,025[a]	1,847	1,023–2,178[a]
Scanning, concurrent	1,199	959	240
Training	1,690–2,536[a]	169–253[a]	1,521–2,283[a]
CPOE support	[a]	0	[a]

[a]Serve as a disclaimer size. (This is an illustrative model. Since hospitals and health systems have unique mixes of local and corporate support, each hospital should carefully develop their specific model based on their resources.)

primary support for all staff and physicians who interact within their unit/department, and utilize their informatics resources as secondary (second tier) support.

One guiding principle is that each facility must have adequate training and support personnel to be completely successful with the preparation, activation, and ongoing support of all staff and physicians under CPOE processes. CPOE activations should primarily rely on local resources for front-line support of the medical staff and employees. The CPOE team should provide additional support for each facility. These persons should support the local front-line support team (trainers and facility Super-Users) from 6 weeks prior to activation through the first month of go-live support. Additional IT support should be available for the first few days of CPOE activation to provide application and end-user device/infrastructure support.

The facility should project the support hours based on the number of nursing units and number of active physicians. The author recommends that the facility tracks CPOE support hours within a separate cost center to avoid affecting operational unit/departmental productivity numbers. Once the facility determines the hours of support, they should multiple those hours by a blended hourly rate for the hospital. If they anticipate these hours to be overtime hours, the estimation should include a multiplier (such as 1.5 times in the U.S., for time and a half) to determine cost.

For the deployment model that the author recommends in this book, Table 8.1 illustrates the estimates for hospitals ranging in size from 30 to 350 inpatient beds.

For the Training hours, the facility Training Champion should determine hours of training per role and number of employees/physicians in each role. For the CPOE Support line item, one should estimate that you will need one dedicated Super-User to support each unit/department per 42 h of operation for 14 days. Then one would decrease Super-User support for 6 additional weeks to 25 % of the first 2 weeks. This means that the Super-User would return to 75 % of his normal workload while still having some available bandwidth to support his peers. The informatics and IT team should remain dedicated support for the first 2 months of implementation.

8.2   Estimating Physician Liaison(s) to Support CPOE

In addition to Super-User support for the CPOE activation, the author has created a model for the number of individuals necessary for ongoing support of the Medical Staff. These numbers alone do not recognize additional staff that a hospital needs

Table 8.2 Recommended physician liaisons needed to support providers and office staff by daily census adjusted by number of active providers on staff

	Average daily census					
Active providers	**<50**	**51–100**	**101–150**	**151–200**	**201–300**	**>300**
<30	1	1	1	1	2	2
31–60	1	2	2	2	2	2
61–100	2	2	2	2	3	3
101–150	2	2	3	3	3	3
151–200	2	3	3	3	4	4
201–300	3	3	4	4	4	5
301–400	3	3	4	4	5	5
>400	3	4	4	5	5	6

for the first month of implementation, but rather the post-implementation support. These individuals must support physician office staff, train and support new physicians to the staff, provide ongoing coaching to providers struggling with CPOE and electronic documentation, as well as new initiatives and optimization efforts. The author, over the past decade, has used Table 8.2 above as a successful guide for estimating the number of physician liaisons for a hospital, based on the number of inpatient beds and the number of active medical staff. Hospital teams supporting larger than 500 beds and more than 400 active providers (or separated into multiple buildings) would need to adjust the model based on their needs.

For the purpose of this calculation, the author defines active providers as physicians and physician extenders who provide ED, inpatient, observation, outpatient surgery care or consultation during a typical week (or at least an average >4.5 encounters per month). He recommends that physician liaisons should be salaried, and provide phone support nights and weekends. They should be available daily on the units to assist rounding physicians as well as train and orient all new members of the medical staff. Multi-campus facilities should have at least one liaison per campus. Once CPOE is live, facilities may decide to utilize the bandwidth of hospital unit clerks to serve as supplemental members of the physician liaison team.[1] Without such a benchmark, we often see hospitals underestimate the number of physician support persons. This under-support often leads to physician inefficiency and frustration. The larger risk, however, is the erosion of trust between the medical staff and the executive team if the former feel that the latter are under-supporting their efforts.

8.3   Characteristics of a Successful Physician Liaison

A very unfortunate pitfall occurs when a hospital hires the wrong person to fill the physician liaison role. One should view the physician liaison role as very important and hire personnel who have a gift for teaching yet be able to maintain accountabil-

---

[1] Hospital unit clerks spend 40–60 % of their time with order entry and processing/faxing prior to CPOE. Consider using this bandwidth for customer service activities, concurrent scanning, and/or physician support, though not sole support.

ity among providers. The author has seen successful physician liaisons with backgrounds in everything from hospitality management, informatics, and nursing. However, one should be in his role long enough to understand hospital culture and physician workflows. Therefore, a person from outside the hospital workforce will need a longer time to prepare as a physician support resource. Unfortunately, the author has also seen hospitals hire individuals into this role with less than 1 month prior to implementation and with no prior hospital exposure.

In addition, these individuals must have incredible physical and emotional stamina, as they often must respond quickly into a situation full of turmoil and conflict.

Some general qualities of the physician liaison include:

- Proactive and self-starter
- Able to work in a stress environment
- Active listening skills to fully understand and interpret what the providers are saying
- Ability to explain, support and follow recommended best-practice workflows
- Have an excellent rapport with the medical staff
- Have flexible work-hours including ability to support nights and weekends as needed

In addition, these individuals must be fully competent in the use of the EMR for all provider workflows and have tips and tricks readily available to create innovative solutions to specific physician needs. We also recommend that they be proficient in the hospital's office applications such as Microsoft Office (Outlook, Word, Excel, PowerPoint and Visio) or equivalent.

The author recently had an experience, which exemplifies the value of having the right person in the role of physician liaison. Judi Reed, a nurse that works on the author's Medical Informatics team, recently had a physician who was complaining, soon after activation (from a mainly paper-based hospital to full EMR and CPOE activation), that a nurse was slow in taking a telephone order, entering it and reading it back. Judi looked him in the eye, and calmly said, "Well you do understand, that nurses had to learn how to do **their** jobs as well as the physician's job with this implementation." This disarmed the physician and gave him a new perspective on his interactions with the nurses. A less experienced person may have joined the doctor's criticism of the nurse, and missed a tremendous opportunity to promote mutual understanding and teamwork.

8.4 Care and Training of Your Physician Liaison(s)

Since physician liaisons become critical resources during the implementation and ongoing support of CPOE and electronic documentation, it is important that the organization invest in the training and ongoing growth of these individuals. Otherwise, the organization may not realize the full value of these provider support specialists. Since these individuals are not physicians, they need skills that will improve their success at provider engagement. At the start, they need to be trained in how the EMR works and the mechanics of CPOE and electronic documentation. Moreover, they need specific coaching on how to lead physicians through change. Through the years we have seem many organizations that seem to concentrate on the skills of EMR use without the art (and skills) of physician engagement.

Just as the author discussed in the prior chapters in regards to physicians, it is important that you expose the physician liaisons to the same messages that help promote successful change. They will function at a higher level if they understand the organization's vision for CPOE as well as the strategic IT roadmap. They need to understand the day-in-the-life of a physician, and the responsibilities that they have for patient care. They need to understand the lingo, such as the difference between various documents (History and Physical, Consultation Report, Progress Note, Operative Report and Discharge Summary), various orders (IV fluids, medications, tests, studies, and patient care), and different roles (attending versus consulting physician). We also expose physician liaisons to the evidence and data behind CPOE.

As physician liaisons begin to grasp the basics of the EMR and CPOE processes, one begins to add specific "tips and tricks." These are personal settings or quick wins which may benefit some physicians, but not to the point of being standard settings. One finds it valuable to have the physician liaisons communicate these personally to physicians, as it helps to establish them with the medical staff as a "go-to" person who provides specific value.

One should invest time in helping the physician liaison understand best practice workflows to help the doctors be more efficient in activities such as admission, discharge and medication reconciliation. You should also update them on changes within the industry that will affect physicians and hospitals, such as Value-based Purchasing, National Hospital Quality Measures, Meaningful Use and declining reimbursement models. Ultimately, it is about investing in these individuals to arm them with the skills and information that will help them be successful support for the medical staff.

8.5 Shields and Phasers

As you execute on your CPOE journey, you will have many missteps at multiple levels within the organization and opportunities to recover from those missteps. Therefore, it is important for team members, at every level of the organization, know that senior leadership has their backs. One of the author's mentors, Scott Pittman, uses an analogy from the Star Trek[2] universe: shields and phasers. Scott (paraphrased by the author) explains it as follows:

> "Every person has certain skills, knowledge and abilities (phasers) that they bring daily to their role and allow them to be successful. Each person is responsible for keeping their

---

[2] Star Trek was created by Gene Roddenberry and is a copyright of CBS Studios, Inc.

phasers in prime working order and in continuing to improve them. Your phasers are the offensive tools that allow one to be successful."

"Shields, however, are your defensive tools, that allow you to take a few blows along the way without allowing total destruction during your missteps. However, in the course of human interaction, one will get into a situation in which one will need more protection than your own shields can provide. Therefore, it is imperative that you have the ("air") support of a senior leader who will be your shield when it is necessary. And once you lose that shield, you become more vulnerable to danger."

The author likes to promote to both his staff and the facility physician liaisons that they are responsible for the maintenance and upkeep of their phasers through personal growth, obtaining new skills, and enhancing their skills. They also need to foster their relationships among leadership and create ever-increasing value within the organization. When they find themselves in conflict, they can then turn to their mentor (shield) and determine a course of action toward repair and resolution. The mentor should not merely rescue the person, but rather help lead the person to a workable solution. If a person supporting physicians through the adoption of CPOE never finds himself in a situation of conflict, then he may not be in the front line actually facilitating change.

In a multi-hospital situation, a CEO may occasionally request, to a leader that you remove a corporate support person due to some perceived instance of conflict with a single physician. The leader should see this as an immediate opportunity to mentor that employee to solve the conflict and repair the damage. The consequences of the employee not successfully repairing the situation will otherwise result in the employee losing all credibility at other hospitals as well. Therefore, it is critical that the leader determine if the grievance can only result in the termination of the employee's role. For failing at one facility will often taint the employee across the health system. Without resolution and repair of physician conflict, it becomes a rare employee, whom a hospital CEO removes, who can succeed elsewhere in the company. Most physician conflicts actually abate over time if the participants allow.

8.6   Watering Down Medical Decision-Making

As discussed in Sect. 1.1, automating broken processes get you to the wrong place quicker. This becomes very evident whenever we continue to allow non-providers to accomplish physician workflow. There are endless examples, but one can start with a couple to make a point.

The first would be the maintenance of the Problem List and of Allergies. Once you activate CPOE, both problems and allergies are critical data/information that can drive more effective CDS (clinical decision support). However, many organizations allow non-licensed employees to access and update these tables. Alternatively, they may allow free-text (i.e. non-codified/non-structured) data entry into these areas of the chart. The potential patient safety cost can be huge. For example, physicians, nurses and pharmacists rely on CDS to catch allergies, serious drug-drug interactions or potential drug-diagnoses mismatch. On first glance, an allergy table may appear properly up-to-date, yet be unable to function due to a free-text entry. Secondly, there is a significant difference between allergies and side effects in the EHR. Codeine is a common example. Many patients claim they are allergic to codeine and state the reason that it upsets their stomach. This is clinically a side effect and not an allergy. The right thing for a physician to do is not prescribe oral codeine to the patient. However, this is not a reason to avoid all opioid (e.g. narcotics) medications by any route. Therefore, non-clinical employees entering codeine inappropriately as an allergy result in one of two unintended consequences for the patient: avoidance of all narcotic pain medications by the doctor, or the annoyed physician overriding a class alert and giving the medication regardless. In this case, it would be helpful to have the codeine reaction accurately codified in the chart as a side effect and not alert the doctor ordering injectable opioids.

Similar issues arise if non-physicians maintain problem lists. A non-provider may indicate that the patient has diabetes, while a physician ordering renal-excreted medication may prescribe quite differently if the patient has diabetes with renal complications.

Finally, the use of scribes and rounding nurses, which have been helpful in the office practices of highly specialized physicians such as ophthalmologists are starting to find their way into Emergency Departments and hospitals. Health systems and hospitals have a responsibility to restrict the scope of practice of such non-providers and ensure that they are not performing medical decision-making. As physicians become more efficient with electronic medical records, they will begin to see these individuals as unnecessary expenses, which only delay medical decision-making and get between the physician and the patient.

8.7   The Impaired/Disruptive Physician

To play on the words of an old adage about money, the author likes to remind peers, "CPOE is neither good nor bad, but does magnify who you are." While many physicians may voice concerns about the change of CPOE, an occasional physician becomes quite disruptive and even to the point of threatening. In the author's experience, however, he tends to find that physicians who are disruptive during CPOE activation have a long history of being disruptive at the hospital on prior occasions. Therefore, we would remind leaders that disruptive physicians usually have unaddressed issues that might become magnified during a CPOE project/activation. In many cases, their behavior often becomes a therapeutic cry for help. Rather than face disruption during CPOE activation, we recommend that the medical staff deal with these individuals proactively. Often these physicians are quite relieved when their colleagues reach out to them in their time of need.

8.8 The Slow-Adapting Physician

During CPOE training, the team may note a physician who falls behind in class or shows signs of frustration. Excluding the known disruptive physician above, this may be the first clue that the physician has a fear of computers, a lack of basic computer skills, or even an unrecognized learning disorder. The team should remember that this is not an issue of intelligence or attitude, and respond in a respectful, nonjudgmental fashion. It is important for the training team to identify these physicians early and provide additional hands-on one-on-one training in an environment of safety and respect. In most cases, the experienced teacher can overcome these barriers and help the physician become competent and efficient with the system. The training team should be prepared to offer the same opportunity for personalized training to any employee as well.

8.9 "I'll take my business and go elsewhere" Physician

A rare hospital does not have this physician on staff prior to CPOE. Moreover, it is likely to be a physician who brings significant volume to the hospital. The executive team needs to decide up front if patient safety or physician preference is the highest value. If the former, they will stand their ground with the physician and respectfully wish them well at the competitor hospital. In 12 years, the author can count on one finger the number of physicians who make this a permanent move. However, the author has seen a couple physicians who were already determined to leave and utilize CPOE as cover for a business or disciplinary reason for leaving.

8.10 Blaming the EMR for All Problems

Multi-person access to the patient record and electronic tools can provide staff and physicians new opportunities for efficiency and patient safety. However, sites should fully analyze issues and mishaps that staff and physicians attribute to CPOE or the EMR and determine the true root cause of the mishap. For example, physicians may be making clinical decisions about patient care when the latest vital signs are on a paper in someone's pocket rather than recorded electronically. Additionally we see errors that the author likes to refer to as the CPOE WNL error. While healthcare has traditionally used the abbreviation WNL to convey that a test is "within normal limits", the transparency of CPOE and the EHR often demonstrates that staff/physicians miss critical data/information because "we never looked." Electronic records produce new levels of accountability and transparency of the hospital processes and thereby create new opportunities to improve patient care and safety. However, one must consider all our systems and staff, not just the EMR, as you strive to improve and transform our organizations. The hospital can combat this by providing designated auditors during activation to ensure that end-users adopting new processes are not creating errors of omission.

8.11 Missing the Opportunity to Drive Performance Improvement

Through the years, the author has seen organizations invest in CPOE yet fail to invest in the reporting tools that will provide business and clinical intelligence as a result. Fortunately, AHS has been on the forefront of data/information transparency with dashboards and clinical reporting. They have developed dashboards that measure rates for physician-entered orders, medication orders, electronic notes, and evidence-based order sets. The system updates data nightly and allows one to display health system totals, hospital totals, and down to the individual provider level. Recently they added a similar dashboard to display physician actions in response to specific clinical decision alerts.

In addition, the author likes to monitor end-user CPOE accuracy during the first 14 days of CPOE activation. He instructs the team to look for nurses who put orders into the system as written (rather than verbal/phone, or protocol) as well as physicians who are placing more than 20 % verbal/phone orders. It is important for the team to have these queries and reports ready prior to activation and have a team responsible to review the activation data daily and work with end-users to correct behaviors before they become habits.

8.12 Giving Some End-Users a Pass on Training

Occasionally we have seen some behavior in which the training team will not hold certain individuals to complete full training prior to the activation. The typical reason is that "he is too busy" or "she has already done CPOE at another hospital." Through the last decade, the author has seen this play out at activation with end-users who do not know how to perform their roles, and if physicians, may compromise patient safety. He has also discovered users that allow others to complete part of their computer-based learning modules or online competency modules, rather than reviewing the material themselves. A warning sign is a user, who at activation does not display even the basic skills of CPOE. They typically criticize the project with words and abnormal behavior.

The author recommends that you carefully monitor online training and identify aberrancies such as the user who completes modules in record times or who repeatedly take the competency modules without evidence of taking the online course, as they report, "I watched it with _____." It is best that the training team identify these individuals during the training phase, and remedy the situation prior to the day of activation. Nevertheless, always remember, the person who cheats on training has exposed a clue about his character.

8.13 Having Adequate Devices at Activation

Long before the CPOE go live date, the team should determine the number of devices needed on each unit/department to allow staff and physicians to access the EMR and do their job. In recent years, the author's CPOE teams have done this with a device walk-through that looks at current infrastructure. The survey considers desktop computers, mobile computers, printers and scanners. Ultimately, the team turns this into a report outlining all existing and future devices. As the author mentioned in an early chapter, a hospital will have to postpone activation if adequate number of devices are not available for the staff.

The team doing the survey must include clinical and technical resources. The clinical leadership also must determine in advance if CPOE will bring any changes to the clinical practice model. For example, will nurses use workstations on wheeled carts, or use stationery devices in each patient room. Will technicians enter data using devices at bedside or use special collection devices with an interface to the patient's EHR. Will HIM (health information management) staff scan paper documentation on the unit or after the patient's discharge?

The team also recognizes specific end-users that must be fully mobile for CPOE. The best example of this is the anesthesia department. The author recommends a high-impact laptop for each anesthesia provider. These providers, especially the physicians (anesthesiologists), are highly mobile and need immediate access to real-time surgical schedules and patient information. During the survey, the technical team should note current access points (wireless capacity versus network ports) and power outlets. In several cases, the team has identified units and departments that had more devices than they actually needed to perform their duties. In these cases, the team redeploys the devices to another location.

The team compiles their report and presents it to the hospital leadership to make sure that they address all questions and concerns. Ultimately, the front-end of the process is not complete until the leadership approves the capital and one places the equipment order. However, this is not the completion of the exercise.

Once the equipment arrives, the technical team must install each device; ensure power, and network connections on each. We also recommend 2–3 weeks prior to activation that a dedicated team do a final walk-through to ensure that each device properly works. This includes the team testing the functionality and network connection of each device as well as proper printing and scanning functions. AHS made this a critical requirement of the final CPOE Go/No Go decision.

Despite all the planning, the team should have a few additional mobile devices available as well as keyboard and mouse replacements for the day of activation.

One should remember that end-users spend additional time on a device during the first few days of activation, which may create some perception of temporary shortages. The author usually recommend that a facility solve this by temporarily using a few of their training computers to supplement their devices for the first week if necessary.

8.14   Ensuring Physician Remote Access

Physician remote access becomes a requirement once a hospital activates CPOE. The team should assess how many physicians regularly access your EMR remotely prior to CPOE and estimate needs once you activate CPOE. Surgeons, consultants and primary care doctors who admit their own patients must also be able to place orders remotely. If hospitalists provide in-house full-day coverage, then they may not be high priority for remote access. However, many hospitals still have off-site hospitalist coverage. The technical team needs to provide physicians two-factor authentication[3] tools and clear training aides on remote access. The team should make every attempt to have physicians attempt successful remote access prior to CPOE activation. Otherwise, the physicians will claim that they can only phone in orders when offsite.

8.15   Training Physician Office Staff

Physicians, who are not hospital-based, have office staff that the team should train on accessing the EMR. If the office staff can access the EMR from the office, then you have demonstrated that the physician also can. Office staff must have their own username, password, and two-factor authentication process. Office staff members, who are not providers, should not have any security other than what their role allows. Thus, office staff cannot place CPOE orders.

However, it is important that they be able to obtain billing information and reports to document what their providers have performed in the hospital. Often the hospital team must work with office staff and the latter's IT provider, since network services and firewalls may be barriers to successful remote access.

8.16   Leadership Absences at Activation

Since CPOE changes so many workflows throughout the hospital, it is important that senior leadership set expectations for their management team's time off

---

[3] Typically defined as two or more of three security factors: "something you know (PIN or password), something you have (smart card or random number generator), or something you are (biometric, such as fingerprint or retinal scan)" that a user must have to access systems.

around the training and activation dates. End-users will have many questions as they train, and often discover specific "use-cases" that the workflow team did not address earlier in the project. Therefore, it is important that unit and departmental leaders train early and that their employees can access them during the training and activation phase. Since the hospital sets CPOE training and activation dates well in advance, it is important that senior leadership communicate appropriate expectation and holds their management team accountable for their presence and involvement.

8.17 Key Points

- Create a budget early for CPOE planning
- Have a dedicated plan for provider support to your physicians, hire the right individuals, and ensure proper training
- Make sure your physician support team knows that "leadership has their backs"
- Make sure that medical decision-making occurs by physicians and not passed down to the nursing staff
- Manage impaired/disruptive physicians well in advance of your CPOE activation
- Be on the lookout for physicians and staff who will need extra time and attention for training
- Be willing to let physicians who threaten to leave because of your patient safety initiatives leave. However, do not make it personal, but about the patient, as they often will return once these emotions have passed
- Be committed to determine true root cause of any patient safety or employee mishap, and do not allow your team to first blame your EMR/CPOE
- Have a plan on how you will leverage CPOE to drive performance improvement
- Have all end-users complete prescribed training for their role
- Make sure you have adequate and working devices for a successful activation
- Ensure that physicians can securely access your EMR and perform CPOE remotely
- Remember to train physician office staff and use it as an opportunity to demonstrate remote access from the offices
- Executives must set clear expectations of their management team for training and their presence during activation

8.18 Fingernails on the Chalkboard

- **There is no dedicated budget for CPOE**
  CPOE requires leadership to commit a significant amount of staff time and resources for every phase of the project. Therefore, a hospital should anticipate the hours they will commit to the project as well as the capital expenditures that will make for wireless/network infrastructure and devices such as additional

computers, printers and scanners. In addition, they should create a separate labor cost center for activation support so that units/departments have no rationale for cutting activation support in order to affect their productivity numbers.

- **"The computer technicians will support the physicians."**
Individuals who support physicians through CPOE activation must have the correct skills, knowledge and abilities to understand physician workflows and lead them through the CPOE change process. While technical resources may be able to assist a physician with a computer that does not work, the effort should be that the physician never encounters a computer that does not work. Instead, there should be a defined resourced plan on how to help your physicians learn and adopt CPOE processes, achieve personal efficiency and obtain maximal effectiveness for safety and evidence-based patient care.
- **"And we have three persons on temporary/partial disability that will support our physicians."**
The physician support person must have the skills, knowledge and ability to understand the physician's needs during the preparation leading up to CPOE and the mental and physical stamina to support physicians on every unit of the hospital, at a moment's notice, 24 h/day. Physician support is not a temporary function and a very rigorous role. We prefer that you hire the right individuals with the right attitude and skills to be successful in the role.
- **The hospital fires a provider support person because a physician is unhappy with them.**
Leading physicians through the change of CPOE is a difficult role and even the most effective physician support person will find himself in the midst of criticism and/or conflict during the CPOE project and activation. It is important that the leadership team understand that there are two sides to every complaint and supports their team members unless illegal/immoral behavior occurs. If leadership places "avoiding physician complaints/conflicts" as its highest value, then it is probably not the right leadership team to implement CPOE.
- **Nurses are practicing medicine without a license.**
The author has never seen a hospital in which nurses and staff are not involved in some level of medical decision-making prior to CPOE. However, CPOE and its transparency will not permit leadership to ignore this behavior. Every person's entry in the EHR is time-stamped and documented. Therefore, the leadership must stand firm when the team uncovers instances that they must correct prior to CPOE implementation. Only providers may make diagnoses, determine the medical treatment plan, and prescribe medications. While protocols and policies may drive clinical responses to emergencies and defined processes, the physician must own medical decision-making. The executive team should clearly insist this and work with their medical leadership to correct such issues prior to CPOE activation.
- **"Oh, that is just the way Doctor Jones is," as he throws a chair, keyboard, or scalpel.**
Physicians are humans like the rest of us, and susceptible to mental issues and stress. Gone are the days when physicians sit above the code of conduct of our staff or our community. CPOE is a major change in physician workflow and will

often be a fuse to igniting bad behavior on the part of the impaired/disruptive physician. We need to compassionately deal with these impaired professionals and insist that they get the help they need. This may require temporary suspension of privileges or even termination of privileges to get them into proper treatment. No leaders should be surprised if the impaired/disruptive physician uses the impending CPOE project and activation to grandstand and act out, creating a hostile and unsafe work environment for everyone else.

- **"Doctor (or Nurse) Smith is never going to be able to do CPOE."**
  The author has seen physicians who have never touched a computer mouse learn to master CPOE and become great inspiration to others. Likewise, we have seen others who have unrecognized learning or visual disabilities surface during CPOE training. It is important that the training team recognize individuals who need extra training and even one-on-one tutoring and mentoring through the process. The team should have a place designated for such training and provide emotional safety through the process. There is nothing more inspiring to the individual and the team than seeing someone master CPOE in the face of known public doubt.

- **"Doctor Jones brings too much business here and is too busy to train."**
  We imagine that the same leader who makes the above statement would not let that same doctor perform a new operation on their spouse/family member without training. Once the Board of Trustees/Directors of the hospital has prescribed mandatory training for CPOE, leadership has no grounds for allowing anyone to not train. A physician must be able to access the EMR, review the chart and successfully order in the CPOE environment. Leadership must be willing to place patient safety above physician's inconvenience and insist in his full participation. Hospital executives must be willing to let untrained physicians leave active hospital care until they complete their training. However, the leaders should make it all about the patient and not personal, as they often will return once the emotions have passed. However, if the leadership team makes one exception, it will send ripples of discouragement through the organization and open the door to others in the wake.

- **"We missed giving that blood because of CPOE."**
  As we discussed in an earlier chapter, CPOE may introduce new types of errors into your hospitals that would never have occurred on paper. This is why we put so much emphasis on system design and safety. However, the author has also witnessed hospitals in which CPOE becomes the blame for every incidence without proper investigation. We have observed nurses working 6–8 h into a shift before looking at the patient's (EMR) chart and not acknowledging new orders or missed interventions. The EMR can allow leaders to create new levels of accountability, however, this change in culture needs to occur prior to CPOE with the expectation that activation will include persons committed to frequent chart audits and review while end-users are adjusting to the new processes.

- **"We are hoping to reduce staff once CPOE is live!"**
  With CPOE live, the organization will have a tremendous opportunity to analyze patient care data much easily than they could with random chart audits. It is our desire that hospitals thoughtfully plan for CPOE analysis and reporting and create a framework to achieve this. If the organization focuses merely on reducing staff, they will often miss the true opportunities that they may obtain with clinical

performance dashboards and reports. We hope that hospitals create a performance management plan for not only reporting on how physicians are using the CPOE system, but take the initiative to look for performance improvement in every department of the hospital.

- **"We just don't have time to get everyone trained."**
  CPOE changes almost every process in the hospital. Without proper training, employees and physicians will be inefficient and ineffective, and possibly dangerous. A commitment to implement CPOE is a commitment to have everyone properly train and gain competency. Hospitals are highly complex systems, and we should not compromise on proper training for CPOE. Better to delay the activation date, than to allow implementation without all end-users trained.
- **"We just don't have the capital to buy those extra computers! Let's go with half of the recommendation and if we find out we are short, we will order more after the activation."**
  The author recommends that having the proper number of working devices be a requirement for a "Go" decision to activate CPOE. CPOE is difficult by itself. However, choosing insufficient devices at activation ensures project failure. Inadequate technical infrastructure, whether network or hardware, will derail your activation, leading to staff and physicians who will be distrustful and angry. As the old adage goes, "you only get one chance to make a first impression!" The end-users are likely to see leaders who fail to purchase and provide enough devices as insensitive and uncommitted to the effort.
- **"No one told me I have to do orders once I leave the hospital."**
  As the physician support team trains the doctors on how to access the EMR remotely, from home and office, they are also reinforcing the fact that CPOE extends beyond the walls of the hospital. Physicians providing care 24 h a day need to be able to review the patient's chart and place orders from anywhere they have internet access. The team should view physician remote access as critical success factor for any CPOE project.
- **The training plan does not include training of physicians' office staff.**
  Training the physician office staff on remote access is an opportunity to ensure that the physician can access the EMR and place orders from the office. In addition, the physician may proxy a patient list to the office manager to improve billing accuracy for the professional charges.
- **Executives and members of the management teams are gone for the training or activation of CPOE.**
  Throughout the book, the author has emphasized the need for leaders to train early on the CPOE system and lead their teams through the process. The executives walking through the hospital at activation inspire the employees, as do the directors and managers who roll up their sleeves to help with the activation. In addition, there may be workflow issues that leaders may need to be resolve within days of activation, or personnel issues. It is important that senior hospital leadership set expectations early for their entire management team to be present and willing to help with the activation.

Chapter 9
Implementation

Abstract This chapter presents special considerations for CPOE implementations that set them apart from other clinical IT implementations. This includes the key milestones that leaders should expect in order to go forward with activation. It also addresses the importance of chart audits to detect errors and workflow opportunities before they become habitual.

> *The value of an idea lies in the using of it.*
> *– Thomas Alva Edison, inventor*

Now that everyone has prepared and the activation day approaches, the team should have a defined plan how they will implement the new processes. As the author discussed training in prior chapters, he will pick up implementation from that standpoint of staffing and the logistics of the big day.

The project manager should have an activation plan that includes all the steps necessary to bring all systems up that the users will need for CPOE and whatever else you implement at this time. An early step in the activation plan is the *Go/No Go* decision. A specific meeting should occur of hospital and team leadership about 10–14 days prior to the activation date. The project must meet several milestones for a *Go* decision to occur:

- All planned devices, including computers, printers, scanners, and wireless access points, are installed and tested
- All training goals have been met
- All support goals have been met (i.e. all super-users and support team schedules are filled and confirmed)

Once the executives issue a *Go* status, the project manager initiates the final steps of the activation plan.

The author recommends that the project manager document all activation steps as a timeline with clearly defined steps and person accountable for performing each step. The project manager should be clear about any dependencies that occur in the sequence

P.A. Smith, *Making Computerized Provider Order Entry Work*,
Health Information Technology Standards,
DOI 10.1007/978-1-4471-4243-0_9, © Springer-Verlag London 2013

(i.e. the person must complete this step prior to the subsequent step.) An activation coordinator (e.g. the project manager) then tracks each step to ensure completion.

One large task of activation in the hospital is the back loading of any pre-operative orders that physicians have faxed to the hospital for surgical procedures they will perform during the first few days of activations. The team should complete all back loading of these orders prior to the time of activation. Once CPOE is live, surgeons will directly enter all their orders via the CPOE process. The author recommends that you not make this process retrospective (i.e. do not make the surgeons enter pre-operative orders in cases they schedule prior to the go live date.) in cases they have previously scheduled. However, we recommend that the team perform no additional back loading once CPOE is live.

Security changes for the provider positions must occur just prior to the CPOE activation time. If you are merely implementing CPOE, your change may be limited to updating provider privileges to allow electronic order entry and co-signature. However, you may need to update the providers' inbox to allow them to view orders for co-signature as well as converting auto-dispensing units from charge on dispense to charge on administration to better capture pharmacy charges in locations such as the Emergency Department or in the PACU (Post Anesthesia Care Unit).

From the support team standpoint, the project manager ensures that the team has previously identified the resource plan and assigned personnel to all time slots. Resources should include technical support for the new devices, security support for password resets and improper security assignments, pharmacy support, provider support, and nursing/ancillary support. In addition, you should have ready access to persons responsible for clinical decision support (CDS) and CPOE content in case any urgent issues occur. While the support team should rapidly assess "break/fix" issues such as misspelling of terms or missing order details, the team should use proper change control processes to address actual changes to the system.

As discussed in earlier chapters, the support team should consist of two levels of support personnel. Each nursing unit/department should have at least one super user who can assist any end-user, including physicians. Second level support then supports that super user and provides supplemental person-power to any area that needs additional support. Areas such as surgery must have super user support in all functional areas of the department: Pre-operative area, OR (operating rooms), and PACU. The author also recommends that second tier support stay in the Surgery areas and the Emergency Department during the first 4 days, to provide immediate access to the super users in these high patient-turnover areas. The hospital may have other areas needing second tier support such as an obstetrical unit doing 400–500 deliveries per month or a similarly busy cardiac catheterization unit.

Support schedules should overlap nursing unit handoff times and not occur at the same time. End of shift is an excellent time for the support personnel to affect new processes and improve patient care. The author is very excited to walk onto a nursing unit at change of shift and see two nurses reviewing the EHR of each patient while performing their verbal handoff. It is even better if the handoff occurs at the patient's bedside and involves the patient in the process. It also becomes the ideal time for the nurse going off shift to complete tasks and perform one more survey of the electronic MAR (eMAR, or electronic medication administration record) and the orders for completeness as well as looking for critical results and vital signs.

The author recommends that CPOE activations occur on Tuesday morning rather than a weekend day (However, the author still recommends that initial EMR/EHR implementations with or without CPOE begin on Saturday or Sunday when lowest volumes occur). The rationale behind this is that the hospital may have slightly different processes and staffing during the weekend. While one might think that Sunday may be the best day for activation, a Sunday go live typically results in a tired support staff having a second go live on Monday morning, which is typically a high-volume day. By having a go live on Tuesday, the team will have the rest of the week to work through weekday processes. Saturday will also be busy as physicians covering over the weekend typically show up and need elbow support. Likewise, there may be nurses who only work weekends as well.

9.1   Activation Meetings

During the first 2 weeks of activation, the hospital should hold several regular meetings. The super users and CPOE team should meet during early afternoon to discuss issues and concerns and share success stories. The project manager should prepare an agenda for the meeting to create structure to each department's report. We recommend you start with some basic statistics, such as number of issues, system usage, and know high-priority items that apply to the overall project. Then the local hospital lead should facilitate each department through a short report of their area. If any reports identify issues that demand more than a quick answer, the facilitator should place these items on a "parking lot" to track items that the team will further investigate and discuss after the meeting. While the first day or two will usually focus on questions and opportunities, the facilitator will remind each presenter to move to reports that are more positive by day 3 or 4. Most hospitals will need 90 min for the first two meetings then cut them to 1 h by day 3. All executives and champions should attend this meeting daily to take the pulse of the super users and the activation.

In addition, the super users should have a quick meeting in the morning and evening after the change of shift of the staff has ended. This meeting allows the super users going off shift to share accomplishments and opportunities in each area of responsibility. As mentioned previously, super users should be dedicated support only during the first 10–14 days with no other responsibilities. For example, nurse managers may not give their super users any patient care assignments during this phase. The author then recommends that these super users have only light assignments for the remainder of the first month of support. He recommends that super users log their time against a unique cost-center code so that the managers have no temptation to send them home to improve departmental labor statistics. The author would also recommend that only the hospital executive sponsor have the authority to make any changes to this plan during the first 14 days of support.

On about day 4 or 5 of the activation, the author likes to give a talk to the super users called "the safe and effective handoff." Nurses and doctors perform regular handoffs throughout the hospital stay, and they are great opportunities to leverage the online EHR as the centerpiece. For the floor nurse, the handoff occurs as two nurses are doing change of shift report while together reviewing the patient's electronic chart. For the PACU to floor transfer, each nurse simultaneously logs onto the patient's as they discuss the status of the patient such as type of surgery, pain control, and postoperative orders. For the ED to floor admission, both nurses are again online reviewing what has occurred in the ED and the admission plans. When both nurses are viewing the chart at the time of handoff, they are less likely to miss critical information or orders that one needs to perform. Nurses cannot accomplish these types of handoffs when the patient's hospital chart is on paper.

During the first week or two of activation, the hospital executives should be visibly walking around to provide encouragement to the end-users. Through active engagement with the employees and the medical staff, the hospital executives demonstrate their support and commitment to this major initiative. Likewise, the directors and managers should be very visible and engaged with their teams during the first 2 weeks of support. This is not the time for leaders to be on vacation or at conferences.

At the end of each afternoon, the senior leaders and the project/change managers should have a 1-h, executive debriefing to review events of the day. This meeting should also begin with the daily statistics, and then proceed with each participant offering his own observations. The major objectives of this meeting are getting senior leaders on the same page so that they can remove any obstacles as they arise in any area of the hospital. These typically occur during the first 5 days, but may extend longer if the need arises.

The project manager or designee (i.e. issue coordinator) should lead a small command center with a few phones that roll over from a single activation phone number. The super users call this number to ask questions, and to request second tier support. The issue coordinator logs all calls as tickets and routes them to the appropriate person for investigation/resolution. After 4–5 days (e.g. mid-day on Saturday for a Tuesday activation), the hospital should be able to resort to their usual Help Desk support. If possible, all second-tier support persons should have immediate availability through VoIP (voice over internet protocol) phones, pagers, or cell phones.

9.2   Other Activation Opportunities

The Communication Champion should prepare a daily one to two-page flyer, covering tips and tricks based on frequently asked questions and Command Center calls. Every unit and super user should receive this flyer daily and have accountability to understand the information on it in addition to communicating these to the end-users. Many sites choose to publish a physician-centric version as well and distribute through the medical staff office. The Communication Champion should also have a press release available and coordinate any media exposure during the activation.

Despite all the planning, some areas of the hospital will find workflow issues and need to gather end-users and leaders together with the Workflow Champion to resolve issues during the first few days of activation. It is important that both end-users and leaders participate in the process, and then document any changes in workflow. The team should remind everyone of their other successes during the activation and embrace the opportunity to find new, innovative solutions to old issues. Typically, by the second week after go live, most end-users now will have a bigger picture of the post-CPOE workflow opportunities and find the collaboration healthy and productive.

At some activation events, the author has found it helpful to hold an open-house event in which providers can drop by and get questions answered as well as learn advanced techniques. This is especially helpful for common workflows such as admission, transfer, discharges, and daily rounds. In addition, the physicians' lounge may be an excellent place for a physician super user to sit during the day and have serendipitous encounters with providers in a relaxed, informal manner. Other sites have computers in the HIM (medical records) department for physicians to access.

Finally, one does not want to underestimate the power of food and refreshments during the first week of activation. Often the super-users and second tier support are on their feet for long hours and it is important that they have meals and refreshments provided for the few breaks that they take.

9.3   Chart Audits and Activation Metrics

During the first month of activation, the unit/department manager or lead should actively audit charts and monitor processes. On the nursing units, the author recommends that someone audit charts at least every 4 h to ensure that staff are addressing new orders and performing all interventions. In addition, evening audits should anticipate any patient care issues that the nurse should call the doctor early to discuss, rather than wait until midnight to call for a PRN Tylenol order.

It is important that nurses are very aware of your policy around taking physician's telephone orders. Physicians may be in the car coming home from the intensive care unit at 2:00 AM and have to give a telephone order in route. The author hears reports, each activation, of at least one nurse telling a doctor she "could not accept a telephone order under any circumstances without fear of dismissal." Most physicians will not abuse telephone orders. However, they also will feel distrust when a nurse refuses to accept any telephone orders.

As we discussed in Sect. 5.18, the Performance Management Champion is responsible for analyzing the reports and data during the first week of activation and provide daily interventions in areas of need. For example, we would want to report daily the CPOE usage statistics, including the percentage of verbal/telephone orders versus physician-entered orders. The author would recommend that you carefully look for errors such as nurses putting in orders incorrectly as CPOE orders. The author also recommends that you pay particular attention to your orders for admission and discharge to ensure that your processes are working and meeting all regulatory standards. He recommends that the team educate any users who are making errors so that the errors do not perpetuate. Otherwise, we have seen unknowing staff create errors with exponential growth, if they are not aware that they are making errors. Therefore, corrections should be swift and not punitive during the initial days of activation. Leadership should view these as teaching moments. However, managers should continue to counsel staff continuing to make the same errors on a chronic basis and maintain appropriate accountability for correct documentation.

Likewise, the team should monitor for physician errors and perform further education as necessary. Like other users, the physicians have major changes in their workflows and will need help in finding the most efficient and effective methods to perform their role. While you have standardized major workflows such as ordering, admission, transfer and discharge, there are still unique workflows that individual physicians have, and they will benefit as your support team offers hands-on assistance during the first week or two.

The author especially enjoys the ability to work with physicians during these activations as it provides an opportunity to see the EMR and CPOE processes from the trenches. Helping a few key physicians find early benefits and efficiency will provide others with examples that will give them hope and encouragement to achieve the same. Though difficult to measure precisely, physicians will let you know if they see personal efficiencies as well as letting you clearly know if they are experiencing a burden from CPOE. It is important that the support team help the doctors find early opportunities and not struggle too long with the activation.

9.4   Key Points

- Have a detailed activation plan
- Hold a Go/No Go leadership decision once you meet training and technology readiness goals
- Have a support schedule for super users
- Have daily super user and executive meetings the first days/weeks of activation
- Use activation to establish standardized workflows, such as improved handoffs
- Establish a command post/center to coordinate super user and second tier support at activation
- Have a prepared press release to local media and a clear media contact
- Have a daily flyer for tips, tricks and workflows you wish to reinforce with end-users
- Recognize that no matter how hard you prepare, expect to revisit some workflows once you go live with CPOE
- Provide meals and snacks to your support teams
- Plan for the Performance Management Champion to review daily statistics and report and provide feedback if they demonstrate errors
- Remember, that what you measure becomes better

9.5 Fingernails on the Chalkboard

- **Training goals are falling short**
  As some sites approach their go live date, they may not be hitting their training goals. It is unfortunate when hospitals then abbreviate or rush through training just to hit their goals. By getting leaders trained first, the organization will be able to keep employees accountable to training completion early.
- **"We will not say '*No Go*,' no matter what."**
  Sometimes organizations will proceed with a go live date, even when they have not met key milestones, such as deploying all necessary hardware/devices, having a support coverage plan, or having all end users trained and ready. It is better to postpone an activation date than to go live with insufficient training or inadequate devices. However, a well-prepared and committed leadership team will not experience this issue.
- **"We don't have all the devices ready, but we will get them after we are live!"**
  During the first week of activation, end-users actually spend more time on devices as they solidify new workflows on the EMR. In addition, if physicians cannot find devices during rounds, they will be distrustful of the process and of the executive team. The technical team should make sure all they deploy and test all computing devices, printers and wireless access points prior to the "Go/No Go" call. A project should never fail due to lack of hardware or infrastructure. Likewise, the team must confirm that they have completed and tested the CPOE software/build.
- **There is not a separate cost center for CPOE support**
  The author has lived through an activation in which the managers had their super users in their departmental budgets and a few days into CPOE found that 80 % of the nursing units had cancelled their super users on the same Saturday to individually hit their productivity numbers. This is a recipe for failure. One can only prevent this by removing any financial incentives for managers having the super users within their normal cost center.
- **"Our super users should be able to provide patient care and support the activation!"**
  Dedicated super users are a critical success factor for CPOE. When super users have patient care duties, either the end-users will suffer or the patient care will suffer. End-users who are not supported will often revert to old behaviors and work-arounds. And those who have trained to support their colleagues but cannot, will often become discouraged and possibly disenfranchised. Activation is not the time for the hospital to scrimp on support hours.
- **"We will only have the IT team support the go live!"**
  No matter how good your IT personnel are trained, they do not intimately know the workflows of every unit/department. Only a small percentage of CPOE success is about the technology and functionality, but rather about the change in processes. Super users from within each unit know the old and new workflows and can best support and communicate their peers through this transition.

- **No one is actively working error logs the first week or two of activation**.
  No matter how well everyone trains, users will taken a while to master the system, and errors will occur. It is important that the team monitor and catch errors and use them as teaching moments during the activations. If one does not correct errors early, these will become the new processes and more costly and difficult for you to correct later.
- **"We will not hold staff accountable until we are past the first few weeks of activation."**
  As we hard wire new processes through CPOE implementation and repetition, it is so important to make sure we are supporting the right processes. If end-users continue to make errors despite corrective education, it may be the first signs of passive (or even passive-aggressive) resistance. The managers should intervene early to first understand the behavior as it may be that the processes do not actually work. However, if that is not the case, the manager must expect the employee to change behavior and adopt the correct process.

Chapter 10
Stabilization and Optimization

Abstract This chapter discusses the key steps the team takes after implementation to ensure that the hospital is properly using their CPOE platform This includes the team's rigorous attention to issues and their resolution. Then the team focuses on optimization of the CPOE project. Optimization allows the organization to address specific opportunities as they begin to realize true benefits for efficiency, effectiveness and patient safety as they focus on clinical, operational, and financial goals.

> *Things turn out best for the people who make the best out of the*
> *way things turn out.*
> *– Art Linkletter, Entertainer and TV Host*

Once the CPOE activation has passed, the team focuses on two processes: stabilization and optimization. The author defines stabilization as the steps through which the team ensures that the system performs as you have designed it, and that end-users have adopted all the workflows that you have designed. The system is live, functioning, and physicians are entering orders electronically. Optimization occurs after stabilization, and permits the hospital to transform itself and fully realize the benefits of this effort.

10.1   Stabilization

The team stabilizes the CPOE platform through their attention to various elements:

- **Managing resolution of tickets**
  It is important that the team carefully monitor your issues tracking system, resolve issues as early as possible, and follow up with the person who logged the ticket to affirm resolution. End-users, and especially physicians, become quickly distrustful if they call the Command Center or Help Desk and do not get timely

P.A. Smith, *Making Computerized Provider Order Entry Work,*   151
Health Information Technology Standards,
DOI 10.1007/978-1-4471-4243-0_10, © Springer-Verlag London 2013

answers or follow-up. Many times an issue is merely a training opportunity, rather than a system issue. Because of all the processes involved, it is important that the support person listen to the end-user and understand the issue. While you may occasionally be able to satisfy the immediate concern with a short answer, often the second tier support team will have the opportunity to investigate if the unit/departmental processes are working appropriately. The author recommends that the support team create transparency around the number of open and closed tickets, as well as the priority (grading) of these tickets, watching for trends and understanding how the project is really going.

- **Devices**

  During the first, few days of go live, end-users are typically on the computer devices longer than usual as they are learning new processes and content. However, as the first 3–4 weeks pass, the end-users will start to gain confidence, and adopt new patterns of work. While the physicians often rely on stationery devices during the first days to weeks, many will desire to start moving their work to the hallways and bedsides, needing rolling carts and devices. The super users should be comfortable contacting the informatics and technical personnel to have clear dialogue about device deployment. Ideally, the early device survey had planned for this phenomenon and deployed enough mobile devices from the start to manage this. However, the technical team may see opportunities to swap devices between units based on their users' patterns of work.

- **Network**

  From a network standpoint, the most common issue is the density of access points for the wireless network. While this was a common issue over the past decade, it has become a rarer issue. However, users may still discover dead spots within their units or in areas where users previously never worked. These include conference rooms, the cafeteria, break rooms, supply closets, and interconnecting hallways. Users who traverse the hospital, such as physicians and respiratory therapists, are typically the earliest to identify the areas where they lose their wireless connection. In addition, remember, that patient transport with an electronic chart means that you want connectivity along every path from patient units to the surgery suite and the imaging departments. As end-users report areas where wireless signals drop, the technical teams should assess and add access points as necessary to support these needs.

- **Orders and order set content**

  No matter how well your team reviews CPOE content, the providers will have recommendations for new orders, order synonyms, order sentences (or order details) and order sets. The author recommends that sites have a rapid response to physicians requesting new doses and order sentences. However, they should take longer for changes to order sets, since the content team has discussed them in detail prior to activation. A physician leader should be in the approval process for all CPOE content changes, as they may lead to a return to practices that you have wanted to remove from the CPOE process. For example, many physicians have used meperidine as an analgesic while many no longer use it routinely due to a risk of seizures. However, an anesthesiologist may use it as a one-time agent in the PACU for shivering or refractory hiccups, and as a tertiary analgesic agent for patients with multiple opiate allergies. Therefore, the content team may want to include it for appropriate use, while they discourage it from routine use as a first-line analgesic. Analysts reviewing change requests may not be fully aware of these nuances and approve an urgent change without giving the content team an opportunity for full review.

In addition, it is important for the team to have a clear mechanism for communicating content changes to the providers. Otherwise, the team will provide new content and miss the opportunity to promote positive changes to the physicians. Moreover, the teams must always let the requesting end-user know when they have answered their requests for change, regardless of whether they implemented or denied the request.

- **Inbox**
  With CPOE, the physicians should now experience verbal and telephone orders appearing in their electronic Inbox for them to cosign. It is important to help physicians see how easy it is for them to sign off on such orders every day as they start their patient rounds. This becomes a fantastic opportunity to help the physicians sign off on orders in a timely fashion. However, the HIM department should actively be monitoring the Inbox data and seek out physicians who fall behind in records and orders completion. In addition, there may be technical reasons that orders do not make their way into the appropriate Inbox for signature, or that nurses are assigning telephone orders to the incorrect provider. The team should work with the HIM team to ensure that the functionality is properly functioning and that physicians comply with their medical staff bylaws for completion. CPOE, therefore, is a great opportunity for the medical staff to improve their compliance in this area.
- **Clinical Decision Support (CDS)**
  Even though the team invests considerable time in preparing clinical decision support rules for CPOE, activation will present them with many "ah-ha" moments as rules fire inappropriately, or excessively. It is important that the rule owner(s) openly receive feedback on the rules and alerts from the providers and are willing to look at the rule data objectively. No matter how well one plans, activation usually presents many opportunities to enhance and refine rules, as well as new opportunities to provide additional CDS. The important point of the stabilization phase is to measure firing rates of each rule, provider acceptance, and overall clinical effectiveness of the rules.
- **Basic Training**
  Once activation occurs, the organization must offer two types of basic training: remedial training for those who are struggling, and initial training for new employees/physicians to the team. The author recommends that as early as the second week of activation that the hospital have a defined plan and resources to offer both types of training. This means an instructor and proctors are available as well as computers and a locale on which to train. The leadership must also hold the line to the policy that no employee or provider may work in the hospital without documented training and competency on the CPOE system. Hospital

leaders may feel the pressure to make exceptions. However, putting untrained users into the mix will ensure confusion, hurt morale and perhaps even place patients at risk. It is much better for the team to have a plan in place to accommodate training to avoid these consequences.

*   **Workflows**

    Regardless of the amount of preparation for the project, activation will expose broken processes as well as those workflows that the facility can redesign for improvement. As stated in the prior chapter, the Workflow Champion must work with the units and departments to assemble end-users who can contribute on formulating solutions. While the implementation deals with the quick fixes, stabilization deals with addressing processes that are more complex than a simple huddle of super users can solve. Each *ad hoc* group the Champion pulls together may take several days to weeks to fully understand the real issues and create a workable solution. The Workflow Champion owns removing any obstacles and facilitating the process until the end-users agree and implement the solution and determine that they have reached resolution.

*   **Advanced training**

    Once the providers are comfortable with the basic workflows of CPOE, they will be seeking out assistance to achieve improved workflow and personal efficiency. This may be in the area of orders, content, electronic documentation, problem list management, or any other new electronic process that you introduced with CPOE. In addition, they will be looking to improve their performance in the key workflows of CPOE: Admission, Transfer, Discharge, and Medication Reconciliation. Some physicians will also bring their personal computers and tablets to the hospitals. They will be seeking specific help in improving remote access to the EMR, as well as improving productivity outside of the hospital walls. The author recommends that you schedule specific times for physicians to participate in advanced CPOE training as well as bring their devices to the technical team.

The author will sometimes note that certain physicians will commit considerable time post activation to improve their personal understanding of the CPOE system and commit to achieve maximal efficiency and effectiveness. Often times these physicians need personal reassurance that they can be successful with CPOE, though they may have lost some short-term productivity during the activation. He has found it helpful to inject humor and discuss the four stages of learning[1] to help them better understand the journey.

1. **Unconscious Incompetence** refers to new learning, and one summarizes it with the adage, "You don't know what you don't know." The author finds empathy with the physician who struggles with CPOE and is only now coming to the

---

[1] http://en.wikipedia.org/wiki/Four_stages_of_competence. "Initially described as "Four Stages for Learning Any New Skill", the theory was developed at the Gordon Training International by its employee Noel Burch in the 1970s." Also see, "Learning a new skill is easier said than done," Gordon Training International.

realization that prior to CPOE, unit secretaries and nurses were often struggling with interpreting the intent of the physician. The computer, however, shows no mercy and requires the provider complete each order so that someone else can fulfill it. This creates a unique opportunity to help the physician experience the "ah-ha" phenomenon, as to why written orders may allow staff to commit errors and misinterpretations due to incompleteness.

2. **Conscious Incompetence**. Now that CPOE has been live for a few days to weeks, the physician now realizes that he has reached the second and third stages of learning on various aspects of CPOE. Stage 2 is the physician's recognition that he did not learn everything about CPOE and finds challenges in placing certain orders or understanding optimal workflow. At this point, he admits, "I don't know how to do this!" and is open to instruction and guidance. This is also a time to create safety. Safety may appear different depending on the maturity and confidence of the person. Sometimes the author may meet the physician in the physician lounge or other site, away from non-provider users. Others may do fine with coaching on the nursing unit during actual patient care. In the latter case, however, one should use the opportunity to draw the unit super user into the discussion to create a team experience. This builds commonality of purpose and often leads to a stronger unit as physician and super user work together.

3. **Conscious Competence** occurs as the doctor is able to perform CPOE, especially with direct focus and intent. During this stage, the physician is gaining confidence and starting to understand and enact the CPOE processes. The physician's goal during Stage 3 should be accuracy rather than speed. This is the time to promote good process and attention to detail.

4. **Unconscious Competence**. Ultimately, with repetition and time, the physician will achieve Stage 4. This physician may take 21 days or 30 repetitions of a process to reach Stage 4. However, as they reach Stage 4, they should begin to achieve faster rounding times than even they experienced prior to CPOE. The team should view unconscious competence as the end goal for every employee and every provider. Always remember, it is possible for every end-user to achieve unconscious competence with CPOE, as long as you do not give up on the goal.

About 4–6 weeks after CPOE activation, the project manager should hold a post-activation call to review the project results and to document any final issues and lessons learned. If other hospitals will be adopting the CPOE system, then it is important for the project manager to incorporate key lessons learned into the project plan of the future sites. As the team completes the stabilization phase of CPOE, they can begin the process of optimization.

10.2   Optimization

Optimization can take on many forms, so the team must decide up front the definition and scope. The author likes to focus on three goals during optimization: maximal efficiency (of the end-users), optimal effectiveness (of the outcomes) and patient safety. He recommends that optimization be intentional and data-driven. He also like to stress that the CPOE allows a level and speed of optimization rarely possible in the paper-chart world of hospital care.

Optimization begins with an assessment of your current state compared to your ultimate organizational goals of CPOE (and any other aspects of physician automation). The person or team heading optimization should look at any metrics as well as survey end-users for subjective feedback. Optimization ideally should address both system performance as well as end-user perceptions of efficiency and effectiveness.

System optimization focuses on the EMR experience, such as cycle times for end-users. Your analysis should look at system availability (such as percent up time) and response times. Common metrics include mean times for common functions such as EMR log on, order processing, search, and specific launch time of advanced tools such as medication reconciliation and admission/discharge tools. At AHS, the CPOE team specifically looks at percentage of transactions occurring in less than 2 s. The team should look for processes that do not meet system performance standards and work with the vendor to determine and remove bottlenecks. You may need to assess server loads and balancing, CPU utilization, memory, application settings and network traffic. Our EMR vendor is also quite aggressive of using their client base to determine system performance benchmark and to eliminate any non-optimal settings that may slow response times. Remember that with large numbers of users on the EMR, a small change to remove a processing bottleneck, may result in users collectively achieving hours each month of improved efficiencies.

As the technical assessment proceeds, the team should move beyond single processes and begin to look at performance across processes that are more complicated. For example, the physician discharge process is actually a series of processes, which include an order for discharge, a discharge plan of care (e.g. diet, activity, restrictions and self-care), follow-up appointments, patient education and medication reconciliation. Ideally, the team should be able to create reports to identify outliers and variances across users and departments/facilities. The team should determine the benchmark standard for the process, and then understand which sub-processes are contributing to inefficiencies from a system standpoint. Communication to leadership should include a regular report of system performance as well as process toward removing the bottlenecks.

As system optimization occurs, the clinical team should focus on the end-user experience. The team should utilize direct observation and analytical data to address opportunities and catalogue them as opportunities for training, workflow redesign, and EMR redesign either individually or together. Moreover, the team should consider if they know any "quick wins" which will improve the end-user experience with a minimal amount of effort and no detailed training. The optimization team must also address end-user issues around the changes in practices that occur with CPOE. In some cases, nurses may have been doing medical workflow by proxy, due to longstanding community practices or physician convenience. Therefore, efforts at optimization should not focus on a return to baseline practices, but rather opportunities to enhance and improve provider efficiency while improving outcomes and achieving safer patient care processes.

During the optimization phase, the team cannot over communicate to the hospital(s) and end-users. The team should leverage multiple formats for communication. As discussed earlier, the site should have a Physician Informatics Committee, which can help to summarize end users' struggles and prioritize opportunities to improve. We recommend frequent communication via medical staff meetings, newsletters, flyers, and open house sessions in the Physician Lounge. At AHS, they also leverage an Intranet page to post optimization plans, timelines and accomplishments. Some hospitals also find email as an effective means to disseminate information to their medical staff. Like your CPOE project, a Steering Committee can help guide your optimization progress and ensure that you are prioritizing efforts.

In some instances, the team may identify that end-users have not developed consistent workflow or practices to leverage CPOE and the EMR. However, the team should assess the core issue: it may be physician training, inappropriate or complex workflow, non-optimal tools, or simply resistance. Sometimes, it may be a combination of some or all of these. The team responsible for optimization should not assume that end-users just need more training. While there are always examples of users who would benefit from more training, the team should not assume that education and training solves all activation issues.

Moreover, the team should look at optimization as a performance improvement process. One should objectively and subjectively assess the end-users proficiency and comfort with the CPOE system, develop baseline metrics, determine a plan to optimize, implement on that plan, and then reassess through measurement if you have met your performance goals. Sometimes these efforts will consist of the team trying small tests of change, while addressing others with full projects, to deploy new tools or drive new processes.

We will recommend some specific CPOE optimization ideas below.

10.3 Improve Access to Patient Lists

The author has found through the years that the foundation of the hospital EMR is that a physician has access to a complete and accurate patient list. Patient lists allow physicians to access certain patient populations for acute care as well as long-term management. Without complete and accurate lists from which to work, physicians may have to search for the patient and risk the possibility of placing orders and documentation on the wrong patient or encounter. Typical lists include Inpatients, Outpatients, and Pre-Admitted patients. In addition, providers may follow special groups of patients such as those on research protocols, or those with specific conditions, such as diabetes.

10.4   Enhance the Admission Process

Physicians benefit when they understand the most efficient way to admit patients, whether from the Emergency Department, from the office or as scheduled events. The admission process includes physician orders and medication reconciliation as well as the provider's documentation of the History and Physical. In addition, the process depends on the registration process, nurse admission assessment, and the various interventions such as lab and radiology studies that occur. It is important for the hospital to have a best practice standard for completing the admission process, and the stakeholders to all work in harmony to complete the process. Since every inpatient stay starts with the admission process, the team should see it as an opportunity to optimize not only the physician portion, but also the entire process.

10.5   Improve Medication Reconciliation

While medication reconciliation represents a wonderful patient safety aspect of CPOE, the tools are often cumbersome and limited by the lack of a medication history source of truth. Often the patient cannot give a clear and precise list of his medications. Thus, every member of the process, from patient, nurse, pharmacist and physician, has opportunities to create errors and inefficiencies. However, over the past 2–3 years, the tools have become better and more intuitive. Since medication reconciliation is a regulatory and safety requirement, we must strive as an industry to find new ways to improve every step of the process. As electronic prescribing becomes more common to all venues of care, we hope that the resultant audit trail of prescriptions will help patients and their caregivers keep more accurate list of medications. Health information exchanges also may provide valuable clues to the patient's medication list. However, these sources of information are incomplete and far from a source of truth. However, they may allow nurses, pharmacists and physicians to better interview patients in the meantime concerning their current medications.

10.6   Improve the Transfer and Discharge Processes

The author believes that a physician should be able to reconcile orders for transfer in 1–2 min, and strives to see providers perform at that benchmark. The goal for discharge is 3–5 min for all the steps except for the discharge summary. In order to achieve this goal, the team should monitor the entire discharge process from the order to discharge through the patient actually leaving the hospital. Ideally, this should be 30 min or less. Within the physician workflow, there may be multiple sub-processes such as the order to discharge, discharge medication reconciliation, prescribing writing (or electronic transmission), discharge plan (diet, activity, home monitoring and reasons to call before your appointment), one or more follow up appointments, and patient education on the primary procedure or diagnosis. The team should be able to breakdown and report on each sub-process and determine mean times and variances and look for outliers at either end. Through careful study of the best and worst performers, the team should gain insight on best practice workflow and opportunities to redesign processes. Finding more efficient ways for the doctors and nurses to discharge patients create patient and end-user satisfaction and result in a better process for all.

10.7 Improve the Order Catalogue

Despite all attempts for the team to produce a physician-friendly order catalogue, physicians have great variance in what they call things, as do radiology departments and laboratories. There are numerous ways to improve order-naming convention. However, every solution may bring unintended consequences as your order catalogue expands. Through the years, we have utilized multiple techniques to improve ordering speed and accuracy:

- Provide common synonyms to orders
- Avoid hyphens
- Utilize an order style guide
- Standardize imaging modalities (e.g. MR for magnetic resonance imaging, and CT for computerized tomography)
- Use physician-friendly terms (insert foley[2] catheter as synonym for urinary catheter)
- Construct folders to group common orders, such as Common ED Orders, Common X-ray Studies, or Common IV Fluids
- Use order sets to group typical orders for procedures and conditions
- Provide online and printed reference guides to users[3]

---

[2] It is important to avoid the use of brand names and trademarks in orders except for medications. Foley catheter is a type of urinary catheter rather than a brand or trademark.

[3] AHS had a hospital create a laminated chart of common imaging procedures with arrows to a silhouette of a person for quick reference. It had one page for each modality such as CT, MR, nuclear medicine, ultrasound, and standard radiology. Many hospitals made it available at each doctor dictation station in the hospital.

10.8   Provide Enhanced CPOE Content

The CPOE content team should make every attempt to understand the needs of the physicians and provide content for any new procedures and service lines as well as maintaining regular updates to the evidence. Physician efficiency and patient safety must be equal goals of the CPOE content. At AHS, the team continues to demonstrate improved financial, operational and clinical outcomes when physicians utilize evidence-based content over ad hoc orders. They currently monitor the use of evidence-based content on for 13 diagnoses/procedures, aligning this with the CMS Inpatient Quality Measures (formerly the National Hospital Inpatient Quality Measures and Surgical Care Improvement Program, NHIQM and SCIP). Ultimately, the team should be able to understand the use and non-use of specific orders within each order set and redesign them around peak efficiency.

10.9   Improve CDS

The author has had tremendous success at refining clinical decision support to reduce nuisance alerts and influence physician-ordering behavior. Initially he had a large number of false positive alerts and inappropriate duplicate medication alerts for the correct ordering of multimodal insulin and similar situations. At AHS, we saw providers in 2011 make over one-half million, medication changes based on clinical decision alerts on 6.6 million medication orders, which the physicians placed with CPOE. In 2012, we have seen an overall drop in alerts as physicians have become more familiar with CPOE and have better adopted evidence-based order sets.

In 2012, AHS introduced a Provider Alert Dashboard that provides specific data on alert rates, override and physician actions. In addition to providing corporate data on these alerts, one can drill down on the dashboard to view data at the hospital level as well as down to the provider level. In addition, the dashboard highlights any alerts by hospital and provider in which the override rate is 100 % or exceeds three standard deviations of the corporate average. This provides complete transparency to all management teams and providers and allows our CDS Advisory Committee to identify new opportunities to optimize our CDS offerings. The author is most excited about the future direction of CDS, as medication and patient safety are the primary goals of CPOE.

10.10   Improve Electronic Documentation

As AHS rolled out CPOE, the team saw physicians rapidly adopt electronic documentation for both Emergency Department as well as inpatient care. While some physicians are great at concise documentation, some are very poor and throw endless minutia into their progress notes. While colleagues in the industry debate the use of SOAP (Subjective, Objective, Assessment, Plan format) notes versus APSO (Assessment, Plan, Subjective, Objective format) notes, AHS has been specifically training new users to author more precise, less wordy notes. The goal is to create a self-correcting environment in which physicians influence their peers to document more accurately and concise.

Meanwhile, the federal Office of the Inspector General (OIG) issued an advisory in early 2012 for CMS to begin looking to recover professional reimbursement from physicians who copy each other's documentation and then bill for services. As colleges and universities use national language processing (NLP) to read research papers, theses, and dissertations, looking for plagiarism, it is only a matter of time before CMS leverages similar tools to identify "medical documentation plagiarism." It is important for hospitals to create policies on this topic as well as audit against their policy.

Ultimately, documentation optimization should produce digitalized notes that are the proper balance of narrative history of present illness, review of pertinent data/information, codified diagnoses and problems, and a clear, concise assessment and plan. The author also encourages physicians to order from within Progress Notes to produce a daily summary of care for monitoring the hospital stay and improve peer-to-peer handoffs.

10.11   Develop CPOE Dashboards

In addition to the Provider Alerts Dashboard above, AHS nightly publishes CPOE metrics, electronic documentation and order set usage for all hospitals and providers. The author is a huge proponent for data transparency with the belief that what you measure gets better. It is helpful for each hospital administration and leadership team to be able to view their data in comparison to other hospitals and corporate averages. The author suspects that this transparency has helped AHS to maintain CPOE rates at over 87 % for the past 2 years.

10.12 Report Physician-Specific Performance

Ultimately, hospitals should strive to provide physician-specific performance data on quality and safety, in addition to process measures such as CPOE rates, use of evidence-based medicine and behavior toward CDS. True optimization occurs as physicians collaborate with the hospital to support CPOE, patient safety and satisfaction initiatives, and suggest more efficient and effective ways to leverage the EMR tools and the information found in the electronic health record.

10.13 Key Points

- Following implementation of CPOE, the team should have a defined process for stabilizing the system.
- The project manager performs a post-activation debrief to understand lessons learned in order to improve future CPOE activations.
- Stabilization should include resolution of activation tickets, as well as attention to infrastructure, content and processes.
- At the individual end-user level, the goal is to lead the physician from a state of unconscious and conscious incompetence to internalization (unconscious competence) of CPOE knowledge and processes.
- Once CPOE stabilizes, the team can focus on optimization efforts.
- Optimization should address system performance as well as individual performance with end goals of maximal efficiency, optimal effectiveness, and patient safety.
- Optimization should be data driven with both subjective and objective input to set priorities.

10.14 Fingernails on the Chalkboard

- **Post activation tickets are not resolved**.
  It is important for the activation team to address all Help Desk tickets to understand common themes and ensure that the team has resolved their issues.
- **There are inadequate devices available for mobility of the nurses and physicians**.
  It is important to monitor how nurses and providers are using devices to access the EMR. While many doctors prefer stationery desktop devices during the first few days of CPOE, many will eventually move to mobile computing as they gain confidence and competence with the EMR.
- **Users report that their wireless connections drop while performing patient care**.

During the initial activation, doctors and nurses have a tendency to congregate around the central nurses' station. As users become more confident, they tend to become more mobile. As they become more mobile, the wireless infrastructure may not fully support the number of devices in some areas. Therefore, the wireless infrastructure may need modifications as the usage patterns change due to this behavior. The technical team will need to respond in a timely matter to resolve any wireless deficits.

- **"There never seems to be any time to do optimization activities."**
  With Meaningful Use, tight budgets and other new clinical IT projects, organizations may find it hard to commit time and resources to optimization. However, every system can improve, and the end-users who do CPOE every day are a great resource to provide ideas as well as shine a light on broken processes and less than optimal workflows. Hospitals should place importance on optimization efforts and see them as the next step toward realizing the financial, operational and clinical benefits of their EMR and CPOE investments.

- **Optimization is complaint driven**, rather than **data driven**.
  There will always be physicians who detest CPOE. In addition, there will be opportunities to improve the EMR performance and provider usability. A disciplined CPOE team will collect baseline metrics, create optimization solutions and measure the results against the baseline. By collecting system and usability metrics, the team can move from answering and reacting to complaint-driven questions, to proactive redesign created to improve the physicians' experiences. Then, as the team makes changes, they can measure the new state and determine if these changes gained the expected benefits.

- **"It takes too long to do CPOE."**
  If a hospital only deploys CPOE, then this may be a valid physician concern or observation. However, the CPOE team should design a project in which experienced physicians should report shortening (improvement) of their patient rounding times as they work completely with an electronic record and have ready access to patient information. In addition, the team should monitor specific aspects of CPOE processes and objectively identify physicians and other end-users who are struggling with any step in the health care continuum. The team should objectively review their design and determine if end-users have detected any specific bottlenecks, or those who need further education and training.

- **CPOE adoption rates are low** (<**80**%)
  CPOE adoption rates less than 80 % may indicate that you may have either compliance issues or that you have not optimized physician workflows. Seeing such rates, the team may want to look at hourly compliance rates to determine if physicians are giving the majority of telephone and verbal orders during the night, evening, or daytime. In addition, it may be helpful to look at orders during the admission and discharge processes. As with other aspects of optimization, your review of the data will often indicate where opportunities exist for your intervention and improvement.

Chapter 11
Putting It All Together

Abstract This chapter summarizes the key aspects of *Making Computerized Provider Order Entry Work* while reviewing the critical success factors of a CPOE project. The author revisits his Four Principles and emphasizes the importance of bringing the physicians and staff along for the journey. He also briefly discusses the future of U.S. healthcare reform and the importance of electronic health records for hospitals to succeed in the future.

> *The first duty of a lecturer: to hand you after an hour's*
> *discourse a nugget of pure truth to wrap up between the pages*
> *of your notebooks, and keep on the mantelpiece forever.*
> *– Virginia Woolf, author*

When one asks the author to summarize this book, and how to really make CPOE work, he concludes, "While methodology is helpful, leadership is critical." Throughout this book, he has shared philosophies and methodologies that have worked for multiple health systems and for dozens of CPOE projects. From single facility to large health system, each hospital has a unique culture and leadership. The successful CPOE project will have a clear vision, committed leadership, and a process to understand how to leverage the organization's unique strengths through the project.

The author cannot stress enough the patient safety aspects of CPOE. Anyone who has seen hand-written physician orders has a hard time defending their persistent use in the acute hospital setting. Not only can nurses and pharmacists misinterpret the doctor's intentions when an order is illegible, but the delays in life-saving treatments occur every day in hospitals that have not yet adopted CPOE. Moreover, as evidenced by the more than 500,000 alerts, which providers heeded at AHS hospitals in 2011 through clinical decision support, CPOE has the ability to influence the provider to reduce errors at the point of initial orders, rather than waiting and hoping for the pharmacists and nurses to catch these errors[1]. Hospitals who implement CPOE should be able to achieve a 55% reduction in medication errors that are likely to cause harm. Since deploying CPOE, the Adventist Health System has additionally deployed bar code scanning of medication and continued to enhance clinical decision support (CDS) rules which adds additional safety to the medication process.

In addition, CPOE and electronic physician documentation allows the hospital to improve the digitalization of the patient's electronic health record (EHR). The hospital may then leverage the EHR to share information to providers across encounters and even across venues of care through health information exchanges. These tools allow the providers to improve their medical decision-making, decrease the repetition of tests done at other locations, and speed the access to results. Through better decision-making, patients benefit from faster assessment and care. The author hopes that this will continue to contribute to a better patient experience and improved outcomes of care.

11.1   What Healthcare Has in Store

It has been truly ironic that the highly technical United States healthcare industry has taken decades to adopt advanced information technology. Today's healthcare leaders must have excellence in three areas:

1. Offer measurable value and high quality health care services
2. Provide immediate and seamless information management
3. Operate with financial stability and stewardship

While superb information management does not guarantee a hospital clinical, operational, and financial excellence, one may find it difficult to succeed in the early twenty-first century without it.

Healthcare reform and new federal payment structures will drive hospitals to provide value, quality and patient satisfaction. The Centers for Medicare and Medicaid (CMS) over the next 5–10 years have committed to tie an increasing amount of their reimbursement to performance rather than to healthcare delivery. In addition, consumers will require more value from the system. Transparency of comparative data across hospitals will drive the market to those who achieve excellence. Low performing hospitals will need to align or merge with those systems that deliver according to these new requirements. Strong health systems will continue to grow.

While we have reviewed the importance of CPOE and clinical decision support, we have not mentioned the many ways that digitalized medical records provide us data and information that one may then use for performance improvement in the areas of quality, safety, and finances. Much like the author discovered clinical, operational, and financial benefits of the office EMR 20 years ago, health systems need rapid access to information in today's rapidly evolving industry. Moreover, as the industry consolidates, health systems need to be able to quickly assess acquisitions and mergers, and determine the best roadmap to implement their clinical and financial systems.

---

[1] Bates DW, Leape LL, Cullen DJ et al, Effect of computerized physician order entry and a team intervention on prevention of serious medication errors. JAMA 1998 Oct 21;280(15):1311–6.

The author believes that a health system can fully implement hospitals (with their deployed clinical information systems, including CPOE) in a 7- to 9-month window if one applies the principles of *Making CPOE Work* to any large-scale hospital implementation.

- **A strong vision for automating new/acquired hospitals**
  Once CPOE is the way that a hospital does business, any new hospital's clinical information system should include CPOE as a foundation for any new implementation. The author's experience is that physician and nurse workflow benefits from the integration. The doctors' orders are clear, complete and concise and the nurses and ancillary departments execute them quicker. Data at AHS also demonstrates that patient outcomes improve as physicians utilize evidence-based order sets and benefit from clinical decision support.
- **Senior leadership commitment to automate the new hospital with the health system's existing hospital/clinical information systems**
  Most senior leaders recognize the importance of having access to clinical, operational, and financial information to improve operational and clinical performance. However, they also may be involved with other major activities such as business developments and partnerships during the season of implementation. While the author has worked with many executive roles serving as executive sponsor for large clinical IT projects and CPOE, there is a kind of magic when the CEO is out front and leading the organization through the initiative. It does not mean that it is their sole focus. However, when we are disrupting every employee's workflow as we implement these complex systems, the staff and physicians need access to the CEO through town halls and similar events in which they can ask questions and get answers and assurances.
- **A defined scope and project plan for new hospitals/acquisitions**
  As you engage for new implementations, there is a tendency to want to expand the scope of your team's successful project plan and add additional new items to the scope. This is usually supported by the comment, "We don't want them to take a step backwards," or "We want to keep them at the same level of functionality." While these promises are well intended, it creates new permutations of workflows and support that tend to add to the project complexity and the success of the implementation. They become a distraction to the project, and have an impact on the many people supporting the activation. While the author has seen teams actually pull off these additions to scope, they come at a price that one could avoid by scheduling these additional add-ons 3–6 months after your core implementation. Moreover, if that new functionality or application is that important, you probably will want to offer it to all your facilities as well. There are always elements of scope creep in every project as the team digs into current state workflows of a new hospital. The author recommends that you save up your energy to address those surprises, rather than stretch your team to add on some new "emerging" technology that sounds like you must have it to succeed.
- **An executive sponsor and committed resources**
  Often at new acquisitions, the CEO (who needs to be visibly engaged as noted above) often has too many other commitments to serve as the executive sponsor.

The ideal executive sponsor is the leader who has the broadest understanding of the organizational culture and the power and influence to remove implementation barriers. This leader should be able to inspire the team, honestly assess how the project is proceeding, and hold other leaders and the champions accountable for their roles in the project.

- **A defined 90-day readiness assessment including an executive/leadership engagement plan**

  The author has witnessed too many projects in which project teams rush in to get started on their project without taking the time to engage the leadership team and set realistic expectations. This includes understanding the culture, asking for their commitment, and jointly formulating an action plan to lead the project. There appears to be a lot of "busyness" instead of getting down to the true business of successfully managing change.

- **A defined plan for assessing equipment and infrastructure needs and approving purchases**

  With rapid implementations, the team needs an early plan to get an early inventory of infrastructure and devices. Then they need to focus on how many new devices, printers, scanners, network drops and associated hardware that they need to add for the scope of the project. In addition, nothing happens with capital expenditures until executive approval occurs. Typically, the Chief Financial Officer must sign off on this level of capital spending. Therefore, the team must perform a thorough analysis and present a strong case.

- **Rapid collection and review of build requirement documents within the first 90 days**

  Whether you are automating a new acquisition or a completely new construction, you will need to collect all the data needed to build out your database tables. This must not drag on for months. It is important that the team maintain consistent forms to collect this data from the facility as well as providing examples of how they should collect and document the information. Once collected, the team should review the documents for any gaps, confusion, or conflicting data. With good tools, the team can help the hospital move quickly through this step.

- **Dedicated resources to assess current state and perform gap analysis against future state**

  It is very important that hospital employees actually document their current state then work with your implementation resources to conduct a gap analysis against the future state workflows. Hospitals, who do not take the time nor commit endusers to document the current state, usually make invalid assumptions. This then ensures a flawed gap analysis as well. The other error occurs when managers and directors lead the current state analysis. That usually results in process maps of some ideal state rather than the reality of what actually happens in the units and departments. With poor workflow analysis, one's implementation and training will be less than effective.

- **Commitment to train all employees and physicians**

  In order to pull off a rapid implementation, the hospital must commit resources to train successfully all users on your systems. This will include training rooms, devices, trainers, proctors, and the committed availability of the employees and physicians to participate. The hospital should maintain records of all training dates, instructors, curricula, attendance logs and competency records. The training manager must keep all records in case any regulatory or accreditation organization requests them during site visits or surveys. There should be no exceptions to achieving training and competency for all end-users of your systems.

- **Commitment to a super user support model**
  The author hopes he has made the case earlier in the book for using a super user model for CPOE support. With whole hospital implementations, it goes much smoother if each unit and department has a super user that clearly knows that team's workflow. The super users are always at the elbows of the end-users. The second tier support can then provide further application and technical knowledge to supplement the front line support.
- **Attention to metrics to drive strong performance**
  There are many benefits to measuring performance. First, is to understand how staff and physicians are using the system. Second, is to catch errors and workflow issues early, before they become the new work-around. Third is to monitor for improvement. In addition, many employees and even physicians need data to reinforce that all this automation makes a difference to their patients' care.

11.2 New Payment Models

In the near future, physicians will be under new payment models and more closely aligned to the hospital's performance. Pilots are already underway to bundle physician and hospital payments as well as having physicians return their professional services payments when CMS denies a hospitalization. Moreover, more physicians are choosing an employment model rather than private practice. Hospitals and health systems will continue to employ physicians to expand their patient networks. Through all these changes, physicians will find their reimbursement tied to their employer's performance and financial well-being.

The healthcare industry will also see a shift from episodic (encounter-focused) care to longitudinal care and population management. As the Baby Boomers age and the American waistlines expand,[2] chronic diseases like diabetes[3] and hypertension continue to increase and place huge demands on care delivery models and costs. The concept of the Accountable Care Organization (ACO)[4] will shift more

---

[2] Percent of adults, age 20 years and over who are obese: 33.9 % (2007–2008). Percent of adults, age 20 years and over who are overweight (and not obese): 34.4 % (2007–2008) Source: Centers for Disease Control and Prevention. http://www.cdc.gov/nchs/fastats/overwt.htm.

[3] Currently, about 8.3 % of Americans have diabetes. CDC estimates that will grow to 33 % by 2050. Source: Centers for Disease Control and Prevention. "Diabetes: Successes and Opportunities for Population-based Prevention and Control." 2011. http://www.cdc.gov/chronicdisease/resources/publications/aag/ddt.htm.

[4] "The Affordable Care Act: Helping Providers Help Patients: A Menu of Options" https://www.cms.gov/Medicare/Medicare-Fee-for-Service-Payment/ACO/Downloads/ACO-Menu-Of-Options.pdf.

and more financial risk onto those who deliver the care. With this shift, health systems will need in-depth data and information to manage preventive and disease-management services across every venue of care. Hospitals will be responsible for managing populations of people, rather than just the patients who arrive in their Emergency Departments.

As the author has done large-scale CPOE projects, he has observed physicians who are working longer hours for decreasing reimbursement. They have committed years of their lives to self-sacrifice and delayed gratification, while they pursued their undergraduate and post-doctorate training. The training programs taught them to split off their emotions and deal with everything from trauma, death and dying, surgery, cardio-pulmonary resuscitation, yet see every patient with compassion and understanding. As the author introduced through the first Principle in Chap. 1, physicians pursued their medical careers wanting nothing but the best for their patients. However, we have an American society that has the highest in expectations for their physicians and their outcomes. They often expect them to practice tirelessly, with absolute perfection, and threaten them with lawsuits when those expectations fall short.

Despite the published benefits of CPOE, it is not surprising then that some physicians see CPOE efforts with suspicious intent. They accuse the hospital of shifting secretarial and nurse work onto them. They suggest that the initiative is all about money for the hospital. It is not surprising that CPOE may become their faceless scapegoat of fear, frustration, and dissatisfaction. As healthcare leaders, we need to create dialogue with our medical staffs, and help them through the transition; not just the transition of implementing CPOE, but also the shift to value-based, team-delivered healthcare, and complete transparency of comparative data. We need our physicians to be mentally happier, physically healthier, and spiritually stronger to face this brave new healthcare paradigm. In addition, this is why we must continue to design and deliver better clinical information and decision support systems. We all need to help the physicians and nurses maximize efficiency for optimal outcomes and patient safety. While healthcare must be all about the patient, we cannot lose our precious physicians along the way. As leaders, we must show the same level of compassion to our caregivers that we expect of them.

However, we must also delineate medical decision-making to our doctors and end the culture of allowing nurses to practice medicine by proxy. One can implement CPOE to automate how "we have always done it," or take the opportunity to fix the broken processes and transform our hospitals with proper roles and responsibilities. We need our doctors to be doctors, and our wonderful nurses to be nurses. This is an area where we cannot compromise our commitments to our patients. Healthcare leaders need to stand firm in holding physicians accountable to the medical decision-making responsibilities in our hospitals.

Despite our Herculean efforts to prepare executive teams for CPOE success, we still encounter those few who want to return to the old ways of faxed or hand-scribbled orders, rather than help physicians and employees to complete the CPOE implementation successfully. Subconsciously, they may likely see "physician convenience" as a higher value than patient safety. We really need to commit as much, if not more, time to the executive team than we do to the medical staff. Remember, the physicians will eventually master CPOE as they learn quickly, and soon see the benefits for patient care. Executives, who do not hold fast to the CPOE principles for success, will see reasons to let physicians wander from CPOE workflows and commitments. These executives are truly the greatest risk for CPOE project failure.

When one weighs the number and length of chapters on managing the change of CPOE against the one chapter on implementation, you should rightfully understand that managing change and preparing the leadership for the CPOE transition is more important than the actual activation. Moreover, the leadership commitment is always a more critical indicator for success than even the medical staff's engagement. This is why we have included Chaps. 5 and 6 to provide you some specific ways to assess a hospital's leadership culture both through survey and your direct observations, as well as through a tool such as the Denison survey. Leadership remains the most critical step for successful CPOE.

11.3 The Four Principles Revisited

The author started the book with his four principles, so it is only appropriate to end with the same.

1. **Every day, every person in health care comes to work planning to do their best for the patients**.
   Healthcare workers are such a blessing. As an industry, we have so many committed people, who consistently give their best to help their fellow man through so many challenges such as illnesses or surgery. Those of us in healthcare IT leadership put so many demands on our teams to implement and maintain our systems, and place so much change on the end-users. We live in such exciting times, and have so much we can do. In addition, we have plenty of data to confirm that we are making a difference through CPOE and clinical decision support.

   However, we must not lose sight of what drives us all, and that is the patient. Our patients deserve the best we can give them. Moreover, our employees and physicians need the best we can give them. We merely supply the electronic tools. The doctors, nurses, and all who support them, give much of their waking time to treat the ailments, mend the broken, and comfort the lost. They experience enormous change as we implement our complex systems.

   The author hopes that this book has made the case for intentional change management. Much of this book discusses tips and tools to improve your success at engaging others for the CPOE journey. He has shared concepts and ideas that have worked for multiple hospitals and health systems. He hopes you find value in them and can put them to use for yourselves.

2. **Every day, every person in health care comes to work listening to the same radio station, WII-FM ("What's in it for me?").**

As we lead change, we find that people care more about what they want, than what you or our leadership teams may want. Self-interest is a powerful motivator. Through it, we can accomplish great things, or stay right where we are.

We must lead our employees and physicians to see a vision bigger than them. If they do not, then they will not. They need to each see value in CPOE, value not only to *the* patients, but also to *their* patients, and to themselves. If the change we require is larger than the value that the end-users see, then they will resist, complain, and find ways not to succeed at CPOE. That is why we must achieve maximal efficiency, optimal effectiveness, as well as patient safety.

From a practical standpoint, we must help them find ways to access our systems faster, round faster, and enter orders and document with improved accuracy and speed. Our decision support must keep the number of false positives low, and truly add value and safety to the care of our patients. We must be willing to help those who are struggling, and keep our outcome and performance data transparent. Moreover, when we do have users who are complaining, we must commit the training and support that will get them where they need to be, not compromise our values and capitulate to workaround, shifting the medical decision-making to nurses or office staff. We are at a crossroads in healthcare, and it is up to leadership to hold fast. Otherwise, we will not have the tools we need to survive to meet the stringent outcomes of the future. We need our physicians totally on board and efficient to meet our clinical, operational, and financial requirements. Therefore, we must keep discipline while we help them achieve maximal efficiency and optimal effectiveness on our patient safety journey.

3. **Automating broken processes gets you to the wrong place quicker.**

The many ways to automate broken processes are almost too numerous to count. Our first wrong process is poor leadership. CPOE projects typically thrive or struggle based on the abilities of the CEO and executive team. Fortunate for the author, he has worked with many tremendous leaders in the past decade of CPOE implementations. It is difficult but necessary to be the change agent to deliver the hard messages that come with CPOE.

Having the wrong people in the champion roles also produces great risks to CPOE projects. While we have good tools for them to use, we see champions who over-delegate and under-engage the staff and physicians. It is rarely ability. It is more likely a commitment issue; of the time and energy, one needs to invest in these projects.

A similar problem is the commitment to honest and effective training. Despite all discussions to ensure all physicians demonstrate training and competency, we always have a few that slip through the net, so to speak. They show up at activation unprepared, complaining, (secretly fearful), and consume a significant bandwidth of the support team. In addition, if the leadership team capitulates, they run the risk of derailing efforts to get it right. The broken process in this case is the status quo. The leadership team, in rare cases will give in and allow the physician to behave in an aggressive manner with the nurses and the support team. This perpetuates a culture of silence, and soon nurses deciding whether they should put their own licenses at risk and practice medicine by proxy, or move on to another hospital where leadership holds everyone, even physicians, to account-ability for their role. These are decisions that healthcare leaders face daily as well as consequences of their decisions.

Another frequently broken process involves registration. CPOE frequently places a huge spotlight on the registration process as you have immediate access to data on how long does it take from a physician's decision to admit the patient, to actually get the patient into an inpatient bed. CPOE allows you to measure precise cycle times, since every order and event contains a time stamp. Fortunately, this is one of those processes that once you expose it, you have the data to fix it.

Another example is the hospital's process of discharging the patient to home. As we discussed, the time from physician discharge order, to the patient leaving the hospital, should be about 30 min in most cases. However, we have seen pro-cesses that may routinely take 4–6 h or longer. We have given you a vision on how to shorten this. However, without accountability and good processes, you will not achieve the efficiencies.

We have presented many other opportunities throughout the book including the admission process, and improving medication administration efficiency through CPOE. The blessing of CPOE is the huge amount of data that it provides so that we can identify performance improvement opportunities quicker, imple-ment solutions, and more easily measure and reassess our effectiveness at achiev-ing our goals.

4. **Today's problems were yesterday's solutions**.
There is no doubt in the author's mind that we introduce new problems, behav-iors and situations with CPOE. There is nothing as humbling as the "law of unintended consequences." I always have appreciated the great wisdom of this statement attributed to Albert Einstein, "The significant problems we face cannot be solved at the same level of thinking we were at when we created them."[5]

Throughout the last decade of CPOE implementations, those of us who do these projects have identified dozens, if not hundreds of potential pitfalls that you may identify and engineer out of your project, those that you do not identify, and those that arise as payers enact new regulatory and payment standards. The work of the Chief Medical Information Officer and the CPOE/clinical informatics team remains. There will always be some need for new applications, new designs, rede-signs, enhancements and optimizations. Therefore, it is important that you have a framework for support, change control, and optimization for your project.

[5] Although, this may have been a paraphrase of his quote, "A new type of thinking is essential if mankind is to survive and move toward higher levels". Calaprice A, editor. The new quotable Einstein. Princeton: Princeton University Press; 2005.

As mentioned above, there will always be training opportunities, at not only the activation, but also as new employees and physicians join your hospital staff. In addition, as you add new functionality and features or upgrade your EMR, you will need additional training and support for your end-users.

You will also need stringent change control, so that your future changes do not become your immediate nightmares. Even with rigorous documentation of decisions along the way, there always seem to be those "this is not going to affect the end-users at all," changes, that unintentionally and ironically, wreck havoc on the end-users. No matter how good you and your team are, you will be humbled at some point by unforeseen issues.

The important teaching, though, is to recognize the law of unintended consequences and thoroughly work through every change with testing, validation, and careful contemplation. Moreover, when all your great schemes fail and the unintended consequence raises its ugly head, seek to understand what is happening and gather many minds together for problem solving. Resolution of these issues may be more complicated that you think. For example, we often add service packs to our EMR to provide new enhancements or to correct issues, only to find that new problems result. Sometimes the solution is to remove the new code (service pack) and sometimes that is the wrong solution, as interdependencies may have already occurred that committed you to those changes. These systems become so complex that you must collaborate, weigh the options, and move forward with caution. However, you also must be bold and not allow "analysis paralysis" to prevent any action at all. Finally, you must have the discipline to perform your "post-event analysis" and discuss what you learned from the acute event to minimize future risks.

On a longer term, you will need some structure around optimization of the CPOE system. You will need some type of prioritization model, such as giving higher priority to immediate patient safety issues, regulatory mandate deadlines, and issues with immediate financial impact. Whenever possible, you should structure optimization as performance improvement, and ensure that you measure your pre and post states and demonstrate that what you are doing is measurably effective. In addition, I like to always be mindful of a quote I first read in Pat Riley's excellent book, *The Winner Within*, "When you are wrestling the 800-pound gorilla, you don't quit when you are tired, but when the gorilla is tired."[6] Perhaps it is important to share another Pat Riley quote at this time in the book, "To have long term success as a coach or in any position of leadership, you have to be obsessed in some way."[7]

Throughout this book, the author has laid out a specific plan to help you make Computerized Provider Order Entry work for your hospitals, your physicians, and for your future excellence in meeting your clinical, financial and operational goals. He has not approached this from the standpoint of the specific build steps of CPOE, but rather the head, heart and soul that you may want to consider as

---

[6] Riley P. The winner within: a life plan for team winners. New York: Berkley Books; 1993.
[7] Ibid.

you contemplate CPOE, implement, or optimize your current system. He also has stressed the importance of your vision, as well as your team for your project and ongoing optimization of your clinical systems. He hopes that you have benefited from the journey, and will make CPOE work for your organization, and more importantly, for your patients.

11.4   Key Points

- "While methodology is helpful, leadership is critical."[8]
- Each hospital has a unique culture and leadership.
- The successful CPOE project will have a clear vision and committed leadership.
- Eliminating your doctor's hand-written orders and providing clinical decision support provide tremendous value for your patient safety efforts.
- CPOE has the ability to influence the provider to reduce errors at the point of initial orders, rather than waiting and hoping for the pharmacists and nurses to catch these errors.
- Today's healthcare organizations must have excellence in three areas:

   1. Health care delivery
   2. Information management
   3. Financial management

- Hospitals will need electronic health records to meet outcome standards and new payment reforms.
- Transparency of comparative data across hospitals will drive the market to those who achieve excellence.
- We must help our physicians to transcend old paradigms and adjust to new workflows and business models.
- Failure of poor performing hospitals will lead to consolidation with the industry. Subsequently, health systems will need to develop rapid automation processes to take paper-based hospitals to electronic health records.
- Remember the author's four principles of clinical systems automation:

   1. Every day, every person in health care comes to work planning to do their best for the patients.
   2. Every day, every person in health care comes to work listening to the same radio station, WII-FM ("What's in it for me?").
   3. Automating broken processes gets you to the wrong place quicker.
   4. Today's problems were yesterday's solutions.

- Manage the change of CPOE and bring your physicians and staff alongside you during the process.

---

[8] The author.

11.5   Fingernails on the Chalkboard

- **Physicians who say, "I don't need to change," and executives who enable persistence of that belief**.
  We hope that we have made the case, throughout this book, of the need for CPOE and the importance of hospital executives and leaders to have relentless commitment to the process. Executives who place physician convenience above patient safety will find it difficult to mean the rapidly changing landscape of healthcare reform. We who develop and deploy systems, however, must strive to make our EMRs more user-friendly and efficient for the providers who use them.
- "**We have decided to not pursue CPOE**."
  The Centers for Medicare and Medicaid (CMS) and the Department of Health and Human Services (HHS), who control about half of the healthcare expenditures of the United States in 2012, have set forth programs that will likely reduce CMS reimbursement by up to 10 % in the next 5 years. They are planning penalties for not adopting Meaningful Use, for high readmissions, low performance on national quality measures and incidence of untoward complications. Many predict it will be very difficult to meet these new standards without electronic health records including CPOE.
- "**I've read the book, now I'm an expert on CPOE!**"
  Remember the author's comment from earlier in the book, "If you have seen one CPOE project, you have seen one CPOE project." While we hope this book will lead to more awareness and dialogue around the leadership and change management requirements of CPOE, you need experience and a dedicated team who will get you there. It takes a village to make CPOE succeed. However, we hope this book provides you insights and tools to avoid some of the pitfalls that many organizations have faced along their CPOE journey.

Appendices

Appendix A: Roles and Responsibilities of CPOE Champions

- Stakeholder Engagement Champion

  - Identify a stakeholder team to assist with stakeholder identification, analysis and engagement efforts during the CPOE project
  - Lead stakeholder team in performing the Stakeholder Analysis of the organization
  - Develop a Stakeholder Engagement Plan for individuals and groups impacted by CPOE
  - Review and sign-off on Stakeholder Engagement Plan
  - Facilitate and monitor stakeholder engagement activities within the facility
  - Communicate and support the project vision at the facility
  - Participate in monthly champion meetings and provide updates on stakeholder activities
  - Communicate project status, conflicts and risks to executive champion and team members

- Communication Champion

  - Identify staff and management to be a part of the communication team and assist communication efforts within the facility
  - Lead team in assessment of current communication resources and development of communication strategies
  - Review and sign-off on Communication Plan
  - Facilitate and monitor the activities of the communication team
  - Communicate and support the project vision at the facility
  - Participate in monthly champion meetings and provide updates on communication activities
  - Communicate project status, conflicts and risks to executive champion and team members

P.A. Smith, *Making Computerized Provider Order Entry Work*,
Health Information Technology Standards,
DOI 10.1007/978-1-4471-4243-0, © Springer-Verlag London 2013

- Training Champion

    - Identify staff to assist with learning and training efforts
    - Lead in compiling a Learning Needs Assessment to identify current knowledge and skill levels of various user groups, training resources, and training methods
    - Coordinate CPOE training with other facility activities that may compete for resources
    - Review and sign-off on Training Plan
    - Successfully executive and complete the Training Plan
    - Communicate and support the project vision at the facility
    - Participate in monthly champion meetings and provide updates on training activities
    - Communicate project status, conflicts and risks to executive champion and team members

- Workflow Champion

    - Identify workflow redesign team
    - Assess current state processes to determine which processes will require workflow redesign in moving the organization to CPOE
    - Review CPOE protocol orders, standing orders, and order sets to identify changes needed due to workflow impact
    - Facilitate gap analysis with list of key processes impacted by CPOE, including current and future state process maps
    - Review and update the Start-Stop-Continue Document for the facility
    - Collaborate with Training Champion in communicate workflow changes that require specific training
    - Work with Employee Impact Champion to assess skills and competencies for roles with significant changes to workflow
    - Communicate and support the project vision at the facility
    - Participate in monthly champion meetings and provide updates on workflow activities
    - Communicate project status, conflicts and risks to executive champion and team members

- Performance Management Champion

    - Assess current metrics and analytics for baseline and post-CPOE comparisons
    - Identify baseline metrics for physician usage of specific orders/order sets
    - Assist with design of CPOE performance indicator scorecard
    - Assist with development of communication plan regarding dissemination of performance management measurements to physicians and staff
    - Monitor and assess metrics and analytics data to track overall CPOE success and return on investment (ROI)
    - Review daily post-activation reports for compliance with CPOE processes starting at time of go live

- Communicate and support the project vision at the facility
- Participate in monthly champion meetings and provide updates on performance management activities
- Communicate project status, conflicts and risks to executive champion and team members

- Employee Impact Champion

  - Perform Retention Assessment to identify key employees for CPOE project and develop strategies for retention.
  - Crosswalk Stakeholder Analysis with Stakeholder Champion to ensure high risk, high value employees are included in the Retention Plan
  - Review and sign-off on Retention Plan
  - Facilitate and monitor retention activities during project
  - Collaborate with Workflow Champion to assess skills and competencies for roles with significant changes to workflow and/or job responsibilities. Subsequently, ensure review and update of impacted job descriptions
  - Communicate and support the project vision at the facility
  - Participate in monthly champion meetings and provide updates on employee impact and retention activities
  - Communicate project status, conflicts and risks to executive champion and team members

- Knowledge Management Champion

  - Maintain a secure environment for facility's document library, toolkits and metrics/analytics results
  - Follow organization's processes for document indexing and storage
  - Assist the CPOE Change Manager in compiling and posting results from the various tools, activities and surveys
  - Facilitate training of a backup team member for knowledge management
  - Communicate and support the project vision at the facility
  - Participate in monthly champion meetings and provide updates on knowledge management activities including initial orientation of champions to the knowledge library
  - Communicate project status, conflicts and risks to executive champion and team members

- Executive and Leadership Coaching Champion

  - Assess leadership's capacity to successfully implement and follow through on the change effort needed for CPOE throughout the project
  - Determine gaps in skills and/or participation among leadership and develop strategies to address them as they are identified
  - Provide education, training and coaching to Champions and members of the leadership team on a regular basis
  - Create visible involvement and ownership of the project and the management of associated change

- – Energize champions when they need it
- – Communicate and lead the project vision at the facility
- – Participate in all monthly champion meetings
- – Communicate project status, conflicts and risks to champion team members

- Community Champion

  - – Participate in monthly champion meetings and key CPOE project events
  - – Be the patient advocate and represent their interests are these meetings and events
  - – Be capable of clearly communicating the benefits of CPOE to laypersons
  - – Assist the Communication Champion in identifying communication methods and opportunities to the community
  - – Contribute at least one article in the ongoing CPOE newsletter series to share personal perception on the vision and impact of the project for the community

- Physician Champion(s)

  - – Serve on local Physician Informatics Committee
  - – Participate actively on team, champion meetings and project key events
  - – Train and guide SuperUsers before and after the implementation
  - – Advocate for CPOE among peers and during medical staff meetings
  - – Be well-versed with CPOE literature and business case
  - – Communicate and support the project vision at the facility
  - – Participate in monthly champion meetings and represent the interests of the medical staff
  - – Communicate project status, conflicts and risks to executive champion and team members

Appendix B: Example of Knowledge Transfer Agreement[1]

Training Knowledge Transfer Agreement

Training Champion:

Facility:

Overview:
Each CPOE site will develop a Training Plan to outline course materials, class format and time schedules for each stakeholder group in need of training. This plan will include competencies to ensure all end-users are trained to function in a CPOE environment.

Facility Training Champion Responsibilities:

Responsibility	Initial for Acceptance
Participate in learning needs assessment to identify current knowledge and skill levels of various user groups, resources, and training methods.	
Identify staff and management to assist with learning and training efforts.	
Coordinate CPOE training with other facility activities that may compete for resources.	
Review and sign-off on training plan for submittal to the local facility knowledge toolkit.	
Successfully execute the training plan.	
Communicate and support the project vision at facility.	
Participate in monthly champion meetings and provide updates on training activities.	
Communicate project status conflicts and risks to executive champion and team members.	

Sign Off

I hereby sign off on documents related to the Training Plan placed in the knowledge management toolkit and accept the responsibilities defined above.

Facility Training Champion: _____   Date: _____

Executive Sponsor: _____   Date: _____

Change Management Lead:_____   Date: _____

[1] Adventist Health System Information Services, used by permission.

Appendix C: Employee Retention Plan[2]

Employee Retention Form						
Name						
Role on CPOE project						
Year of Hire						
Internal Drivers						
External Drivers						
Comments						
Check point + 2 months						
Check point +4 months						
Check point +6 months						
Check point, End of Project						

How to complete this Retention Plan form
- List Key Participants for the CPOE Project
- Person's role on the project.
- Year of hire.
- Internal drivers are traits of internal motivation of the individual.
- External drivers are other (non-internal) motivators of the individual (rewards, recognition, etc)
- Comments
- Check with individual every two months to reassess commitment level.
- End of Project is final assessment of individual.

The Employee Impact Champion

Glossary

Big bang When one implements new electronic solutions across a hospital, office, and/or enterprise as a single event, rather than an incremental process.

Change control Managing ongoing maintenance, changes, and updates to a system, such as an electronic health record.

Change management The skills, knowledge and tools used to manage the people side of a project

Chief Medical Information Officer (CMIO) Physician executive responsible for physicians and physician extenders (e.g. physician assistants, mid-wives, or other advance practice nurses) adopting the clinical information systems. Typically, he is the executive responsible for a CPOE or physician electronic documentation project.

Chief Medical Officer (CMO) Physician executive responsible for representing physician issues at the administrative level and being a bridge to the hospital medical staff and/or practicing physicians. He often heads up quality and safety initiatives as well as other responsibilities.

Clinical best practice A process of patient care, that you support with evidence-based medicine, expert consensus, and/or proven outcomes from long-term experience.

Clinical decision support Content, rules and alerts, either embedded in an EHR, or externally accessed, that guide clinicians to make proper decisions about patient care. Commonly use evidence-based medicine links, advanced logic, or designed to prevent or mitigate common errors that occur in patient care. Examples include drug-allergy alerts, drug-drug interactions, drug-food interactions, dose-range alerts, drug-lab alerts and drug-lab-disease guidance.

Clinical guidelines Major evidence-based medicine recommendations arising from professional societies/organizations/groups specifying appropriate processes for managing specific conditions, diseases, or operations.

Clinical pathways Programmed algorithms for treatment/ordering to ensure consistent quality and safety in the delivery of patient care.

Community physicians Physicians, who maintain private practices, the hospital/health system do not employ, and work either as individuals or in groups. This is to differentiate them from employed physicians (on the hospital/health system payroll) or faculty (clinical professors, etc., at an academic/teaching facility)

Co-morbidities These are additional diseases and/or conditions, which the patient has in addition to his/her primary disease process. For example, a doctor may admit a patient for pneumonia (primary disease process), but must keep in mind that the patient also has diabetes and heart failure (both co-morbidities).

CPOE (Computerized Provider Order Entry) Some refer to this as Computerized Physician Order Entry or Computerized Prescriber Order Entry. All terms refer to the process of a licensed provider/physician entering orders electronically into an electronic medical record rather than handwriting those orders.

EHR (Electronic Health Record) This is the collective electronic medical records of a patient or a population of patients.

eMAR (electronic medication administration record) Nurses document their administration of medications to the patient online using the electronic Medication Administration Record. Typically, this tool displays doses of medication and their schedule times.

EMR (Electronic Medical Record) A computerized database with one or more user interfaces, designed for the capture of medical records in an electronic, rather than paper, format.

End-user An end-user is any person using the electronic medical record, including physicians and hospital staff.

e-Prescribing The electronic transmission of medication prescriptions directly to a pharmacy by a prescriber rather than a paper prescription.

Evidence-based Medicine Content based on utilizing information from peer-reviewed sources (e.g. literature and consensus statements) to guide patient care while avoiding outmoded, harmful, or ineffective practices.

Evidence-based Practice One leverages peer-reviewed and expert opinions to deliver state-of-the-art patient care, while avoiding ineffective or harmful processes.

Hard-stops This refers to coded, required fields in an EHR that are mandatory, and prevent further action in the patient's chart until the user enters the required documentation.

Hard-wire One embeds content into workflow that will ensure/guide users to follow the correct process with the knowledge to achieve the preferred outcomes.

HIE (Health Information Exchange) Electronic means to allow one to share patient demographics and clinical data. The hospital or entity can transmit and share information/data between disparate electronic health records or for remote viewing by those without an EHR.

HIM (Health Information Management) This department of the hospital manages all medical records.

House-wide As to deployment of clinical systems, house-wide implies implementation to all departments/units rather than a limited or partial deployment.

Lean Process improvement technique (arising from initial work of the Toyota Corporation and Motorola as part of Six Sigma) to eliminate waste and unnecessary steps in a process.

MEC (Medical Executive Committee) The typical name of the governance group that oversees the Medical Staff in a hospital. The group typically represents practicing physicians from various specialties elected by their peers. They administer the Medical Staff Bylaws, Rules and Regulations and operate various committees such as medical staff credentialing, peer review, and utilization committees.

Medical Staff The formal structure of physicians, and physician extenders credentialed to provide patient care at a hospital. Also may include allied health personnel such as surgical assistants and rounding nurses who are non-voting members.

Order sets A collection of patient care orders presented together either in a paper format or electronically.

Path-of-least-resistance End-users adopt the workflow that produces the most ease and comfort and therefore, the least resistance.

Pearls Physicians refer to small teachings or points of wisdom as pearls.

Pilot hospital Where one does initial implementation to test a system/process prior to general, wide-scale release.

Soft-stops These refer to points in the documentation process where the software highlights or notes important data to encourage the end-user to complete at that time. Unlike hard-stops, however, the user may chose to move beyond the soft-stops without mandatory completion of the field.

Stat orders These are orders that the physician/provider indicates highest priority and immediate action.

Super user Super users are individuals that the hospital intensively trains to provide direct support for end-users within their unit, department, or area of expertise.

Unintended consequences Unintended consequences are issues/problems that arise unexpectedly following process improvement efforts to fix a known problem.

Work-arounds Work-arounds are creative deviations that end-users utilize to bypass recommended processes.

Index